Graves' Disease - Diagnostic and Therapeutic Developments and New Therapeutic Horizons

Edited by Ifigenia Kostoglou-Athanassiou,
Panagiotis Athanassiou
and Lambros Athanassiou

Published in London, United Kingdom

Graves' Disease - Diagnostic and Therapeutic Developments and New Therapeutic Horizons
http://dx.doi.org/10.5772/intechopen.111031
Edited by Ifigenia Kostoglou-Athanassiou, Panagiotis Athanassiou and Lambros Athanassiou

Contributors
Chao Ma, Hosam Mohamad Hamza, Ifigenia Kostoglou-Athanassiou, Lambros Athanassiou, Panagiotis Athanassiou, Ruchi Agrawal, Shahnaz Ahmad, Shervin Sharifkashani, Yongji Jiang

First published in London, United Kingdom, 2025 by IntechOpen
IntechOpen is the global imprint of INTECHOPEN LIMITED, registered in England and Wales, registration number: 11086078, 167-169 Great Portland Street, London, W1W 5PF, United Kingdom

For EU product safety concerns: IN TECH d.o.o., Prolaz Marije Krucifikse Kozulić 3, 51000 Rijeka, Croatia, info@intechopen.com or visit our website at intechopen.com.

British Library Cataloguing-in-Publication Data
A catalogue record for this book is available from the British Library

Graves' Disease - Diagnostic and Therapeutic Developments and New Therapeutic Horizons
Edited by Ifigenia Kostoglou-Athanassiou, Panagiotis Athanassiou and Lambros Athanassiou
p. cm.
Print ISBN 978-0-85014-903-6
Online ISBN 978-0-85014-902-9
eBook (PDF) ISBN 978-0-85014-904-3

Meet the editor

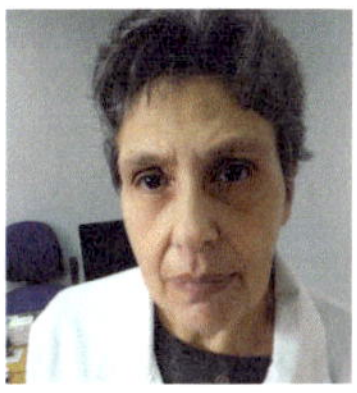

Dr. Ifigenia Kostoglou-Athanassiou was born in Thessaloniki, Greece. She is an endocrinologist who graduated from the Medical School, Aristotle University of Thessaloniki, Greece. She obtained an MD from the University of Athens Medical School and a Ph.D. from the University of London. Her areas of research include breast cancer, neuroendocrinology, melatonin, thyroid cancer, vitamin D, and autoimmune diseases. She has won several awards for her research. Dr. Kostoglou-Athanassiou has published numerous papers and book chapters. Currently, she works as a consultant endocrinologist and head of the Endocrine Department, Asclepeion Hospital, Voula, Athens, Greece.

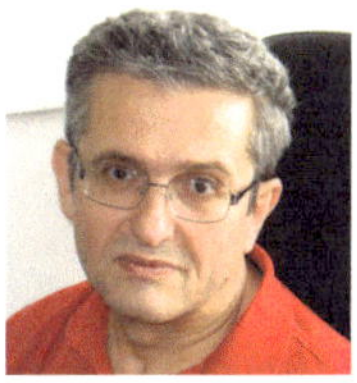

Dr. Panagiotis Athanassiou was born in Chalkiades, Arta, Greece. He graduated from the Medical School, Aristotle University of Thessaloniki, Greece. He is a rheumatologist with a special interest in the pathogenesis, diagnosis, and management of autoimmune diseases. He has won several awards for his research and has published numerous papers and book chapters. Currently, he works as a consultant and head of the Department of Rheumatology, St. Paul's Hospital, Thessaloniki, Greece.

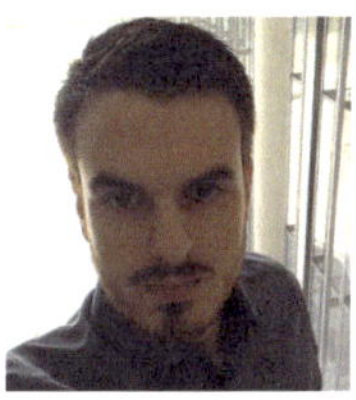

Dr. Lambros Athanassiou was born in Athens, Greece. He is a consultant rheumatologist who graduated from the Medical School of Kapodistriakon University of Athens, Greece. He completed his training in rheumatology at the Department of Rheumatology, Asclepeion Hospital, Voula, Athens, Greece. He obtained a Ph.D. from the University of Athens Medical School. He completed training in the field of ultrasound in rheumatology in Brussels, Belgium. His areas of research include vitamin D, osteoporosis, pain, ultrasound in rheumatology, and autoimmune diseases. He has won several awards for his research. Dr. Athanassiou has published numerous papers and book chapters, which have attracted multiple citations. Currently, he works as a consultant rheumatologist at the Department of Rheumatology, St. Paul's Hospital, Thessaloniki, Greece.

Contents

Preface

Graves' disease is the most typical form of hyperthyroidism worldwide. It is a common form of thyroid disease, and it affects the patient's quality of life as it is a cause of morbidity and, in some cases, disfigurement. The disease has attracted the interest of patients, physicians, and scientists lately, as it is an autoimmune thyroid disease, and its exact etiology and pathophysiology have not yet been clarified. Graves' disease is an autoimmune thyroid disease causing hyperthyroidism. The disease is characterized by the presence of antibodies against the TSH receptor; however, antithyroid antibodies, anti-thyroglobulin, and antibodies against thyroid peroxidase are also observed. Extrathyroidal manifestations, namely thyroid ophthalmopathy, pretibial myxedema, and thyroid acropathy, are observed and characterize the disease. The administration treats the disease with antithyroid agents and ablative treatment, namely thyroidectomy and/or 131I radioiodine administration. The disease may be persistent and, in the long term, may lead to hypothyroidism. Thyroid ophthalmopathy presents a major therapeutic challenge, as it may be persistent and may lead to permanent disfigurement. In mild cases of thyroid ophthalmopathy, the disease may respond to the treatment of hyperthyroidism. However, cases of thyroid ophthalmopathy or thyroid orbitopathy may be severe and need treatment with corticosteroids. Thyroidectomy may lead to permanent remission of thyroid ophthalmopathy or thyroid orbitopathy. Thyroid ablation with 131I, however, may lead to transient or permanent deterioration of thyroid ophthalmopathy or thyroid orbitopathy.

Biological agents, such as etanercept and tocilizumab, have been administered to treat thyroid orbitopathy. New agents, such as teprotumumab, a human monoclonal anti-IGF-1R blocking antibody, are also tested in the treatment of thyroid orbitopathy. Surgical treatment, such as orbital decompression, may also be needed to manage thyroid orbitopathy in severe cases. However, treatment of thyroid ophthalmopathy, thyroid orbitopathy, or thyroid eye disease still presents a major therapeutic challenge. Within this book, the pathophysiology and diagnosis of Graves' disease are discussed. Also, the diagnostic evaluation of Graves' ophthalmopathy and the treatment of Graves' disease are described in this book.

This book is the result of the efforts of various authors who specialize in various aspects of thyroid physiology and thyroid disease. The effort of all the authors is gratefully acknowledged. The great contribution of Iva Horvat for the formation of this book is gratefully acknowledged.

Last, but not least, this book is dedicated to my mother, Areti, whose example and efforts have made it possible for me to become the editor of this book.

Ifigenia Kostoglou-Athanassiou
Department of Endocrinology, Diabetes and Metabolism,
Asclepeion Hospital,
Voula, Athens, Greece

Panagiotis Athanassiou
Department of Rheumatology,
St. Paul's Hospital,
Thessaloniki, Greece

Lambros Athanassiou
Department of Rheumatology,
Asclepeion Hospital,
Voula, Athens, Greece

Section 1

Introduction

Chapter 1

Introductory Chapter: Graves' Disease – An Autoimmune Thyroid Disease

Ifigenia Kostoglou-Athanassiou

1. Introduction

Autoimmune thyroid disease is currently the main cause of thyroid dysfunction. As autoimmune diseases form the modern epidemic or pandemic, and as various factors such as the SARS-CoV-2 or COVID-19 virus are elucidated as being implicated in the pathogenesis of autoimmunity, autoimmune thyroid disease attains significance both from the point of view of the caring physician as well as from the point of view of the researcher. Patients and physicians alike face a major burden of increasing morbidity due to autoimmune thyroid disease.

Autoimmune thyroid disease is broadly categorized into two disorders, Hashimoto's thyroiditis and Graves' disease. In the group of Hashimoto's thyroiditis also belong silent thyroiditis and postpartum thyroiditis. Hashimoto's thyroiditis may manifest with euthyroidism, or normal thyroid function, hypothyroidism, and, in some rare cases, hyperthyroidism, a form known as Hashitoxicosis. Postpartum thyroiditis may present with clinical hyperthyroidism, which may progress to normal thyroid function or euthyroidism or to permanent hypothyroidism. Graves' disease is an autoimmune thyroid disease causing hyperthyroidism. It is the most common cause of hyperthyroidism. The disease is characterized by the presence of antibodies against the TSH receptor; however, antithyroid antibodies, anti-thyroglobulin, and antibodies against thyroid peroxidase are also observed [1, 2]. The disease is a systemic disease with extrathyroidal manifestations, which are a cause of severe morbidity. Extrathyroidal manifestations, namely thyroid ophthalmopathy, pretibial myxedema, and thyroid acropathy, are also observed [3, 4]. Graves' disease may persist for years despite adequate drug treatment for hyperthyroidism. Stress may be a major factor leading to the clinical presentation of Graves' disease. Bereavement or major life events or disasters, such as work or financial loss, may lead to the development of Graves' disease. The disease is treated by the administration of antithyroid agents and ablative treatment, namely thyroidectomy and/or ^{131}I radioiodine administration. The disease may be persistent and, in the long term, may lead to hypothyroidism [5]. Thyroid ophthalmopathy presents a major therapeutic challenge, as it may be persistent and it may lead to permanent disfigurement [6, 7]. In mild cases of thyroid ophthalmopathy, the disease may respond to the treatment of hyperthyroidism. However, cases of thyroid ophthalmopathy or thyroid orbitopathy may be severe and need treatment with corticosteroids. Thyroidectomy may lead to permanent remission of thyroid ophthalmopathy or thyroid orbitopathy. Thyroid ablation with ^{131}I, however, may lead to transient or permanent deterioration of thyroid ophthalmopathy or thyroid orbitopathy. Biological agents, such as etanercept and tocilizumab, have been administered to treat thyroid orbitopathy [8]. New agents, such as teprotumumab, a human monoclonal anti-IGF-1R blocking antibody, are also being tested in the treatment of thyroid orbitopathy. Surgical treatment, such as orbital decompression, may also be needed to manage thyroid orbitopathy in severe cases [9]. However, treatment of thyroid ophthalmopathy, thyroid orbitopathy, or thyroid eye disease still presents a major therapeutic challenge. Graves' ophthalmopathy may lead to permanent disfigurement and, in cases of young female patients, to natural beauty impairment. Despite treatment, Graves' ophthalmopathy may persist for years. Graves' ophthalmopathy is more common in female patients; however, it may present with a severe phenotype in male patients. Graves' ophthalmopathy may also lead to loss or impairment of vision. Pretibial myxedema is also difficult to treat if persistent. It may respond to the standard antithyroid treatment. In severe cases, corticosteroids, somatostatin, and other local agents may be applied. Graves' disease may lead to severe impairment of quality of life, as it needs careful and long-term follow-up. Despite years of research performed all over the world, the exact etiology and pathophysiology of Graves' disease have not been completely elucidated. Several of the pharmaceutical agents applied in the treatment of the disorder are quite old and have been used for many years. However, novel agents, namely biological agents, are currently being tested in the disorder. There is a need for active research in the field of treatment of extrathyroidal manifestations of Graves' disease, thyroid ophthalmopathy, and pretibial myxedema. Thyroid ophthalmopathy is an area where active research is needed so that permanent disfigurement and permanent vision impairment may be prevented. Active research takes place with the aim to prevent or block the pathophysiological process of thyroid autoimmunity; however, these efforts have not yet entered clinical practice. In the book at hand, novel aspects of the pathogenesis and treatment of Graves' disease will be discussed. Some diagnostic aspects of thyroid ophthalmopathy will also be discussed. In conclusion, Graves' disease is an autoimmune thyroid disease that causes hyperthyroidism. It is the most common cause of hyperthyroidism worldwide. The disease is characterized by extrathyroidal manifestations. Thyroid ophthalmopathy, thyroid orbitopathy, or thyroid eye disease presents a major therapeutic challenge and is the subject of ongoing research efforts.

Conflict of interest

The authors declare no conflict of interest.

Author details

Ifigenia Kostoglou-Athanassiou
Department of Endocrinology, Diabetes and Metabolism, Asclepeion Hospital, Athens, Greece

*Address all correspondence to: ikostoglouathanassiou@yahoo.gr

References

[1] Antonelli A, Fallahi P, Elia G, Ragusa F, Paparo SR, Ruffilli I, et al. Graves' disease: Clinical manifestations, immune pathogenesis (cytokines and chemokines) and therapy. Best Practice & Research. Clinical Endocrinology & Metabolism. 2020;**34**(1):101388

[2] Antonelli A, Ferrari SM, Ragusa F, Elia G, Paparo SR, Ruffilli I, et al. Graves' disease: Epidemiology, genetic and environmental risk factors and viruses. Best Practice & Research. Clinical Endocrinology & Metabolism. 2020;**34**(1):101387

[3] Bartalena L. Diagnosis and management of Graves disease: A global overview. Nature Reviews. Endocrinology. 2013;**9**(12):724-734

[4] Walter MA, Christ-Crain M, Muller B. Graves' disease. New England Journal of Medicine. 2008;**359**:1407; author reply 9

[5] Wiersinga WM, Poppe KG, EffraimidisG.Hyperthyroidism:Aetiology, pathogenesis, diagnosis, management, complications, and prognosis. The Lancet Diabetes and Endocrinology. 2023;**11**(4):282-298

[6] Bartalena L, Kahaly GJ, Baldeschi L, Dayan CM, Eckstein A, Marcocci C, et al. The 2021 European Group on Graves' orbitopathy (EUGOGO) clinical practice guidelines for the medical management of Graves' orbitopathy. European Journal of Endocrinology. 2021;**185**(4):G43-g67

[7] Bartalena L, Tanda ML. Current concepts regarding Graves' orbitopathy. Journal of Internal Medicine. 2022;**292**(5):692-716

[8] Ferrari SM, Fallahi P, Elia G, Ragusa F, Camastra S, Paparo SR, et al. Novel therapies for thyroid autoimmune diseases: An update. Best Practice & Research. Clinical Endocrinology & Metabolism. 2020;**34**(1):101366

[9] Jefferis JM, Jones RK, Currie ZI, Tan JH, Salvi SM. Orbital decompression for thyroid eye disease: Methods, outcomes, and complications. Eye (London). 2018;**32**(3):626-636

Chapter 2

Pathophysiology of Graves' Disease

Hosam Mohamad Hamza

Abstract

Graves' disease or toxic diffuse goiter is an autoimmune thyroid disorder. It represents the most common cause of hyperthyroidism. In patients with this disorder, the synthesis of autoantibodies directed at thyroid antigens by specific B lymphocytes enhances inappropriately high secretion of thyroid hormones, thyroxine (T4), and 3,5,3′-triiodothyronine (T3) as well as thyroidal hyperplasia. Although Graves' disease is widely recognized, much ignorance about the nature and underlying biology of this disorder exists. Going through the underlying pathophysiology of this autoimmune disease will reveal how the disease comes to life and will open our vision into new horizons in the treatment of such a condition.

Keywords: Graves' disease, autoimmunity, hyperthyroidism, thyrotoxicosis, B lymphocytes, autoantibodies

1. Introduction

Systemic manifestations of Graves' disease (GD)—the most common cause of hyperthyroidism—primarily affect the heart, skeletal muscles, eyes, skin, bone, and liver [1]. Physicians of all specialties should be aware of these manifestations, as early diagnosis of the disease prevents much of the morbidity and mortality noticed in neglected cases.

It is an organ-specific autoimmune disease, commonly seen in patients with a positive family history, with monozygotic twins more commonly affected than dizygotic twins. It may be precipitated by environmental factors like stress, smoking, infection, iodine exposure, and postpartum, as well as after highly active antiretroviral therapy (HAART) due to immune reconstitution [2].

It is widely recognized that autoimmune diseases tend to be more common in females than in males. GD is not an exception, with women being six to eight times more likely to develop the condition than men. GD typically manifests between the ages of 30 and 50, indicating that age-related factors and hormonal changes may play a role in increasing susceptibility. However, the molecular mechanisms responsible for this gender disparity, as seen in many autoimmune diseases, remain unclear and require further investigation [3].

2. Risk factors for GD

2.1 Genetic factors

A family history of GD is recognized as a significant risk factor. Structural equation modeling has revealed that approximately 79% of the risk for developing GD can be attributed to genetic heritability [4], while environmental factors account for the remaining 21% [5]. This genetic predisposition may also help explain the observed ethnic differences in GD prevalence [6].

The predisposition to GD appears to be polygenic [7]. Several autoimmune thyroid disease susceptibility genes are considered to be linked to GD, including *CD40*, *CTLA-4*, the thyroglobulin gene (*TG*), the thyroid-stimulating hormone (TSH) receptor gene (*TSHR*), *PTPN22*, *FOXP3*, *CD25*, and *VDR*. The *RNASET2-FGFR1OP-CCR6* region at 6q27 and an intergenic region at 4p14 have also been associated with the disorder [8–11]. Genes correlated with the risk of GD, about 70% with known effect, are implicated in T cell function; this indicates the importance of T lymphocytes in autoimmune thyroid disease (AITD) pathogenesis [12, 13].

2.2 Endogenous factors

GD predominantly affects females, and the frequent occurrence of estrogen receptor ESR2 polymorphisms in GD suggests that estrogen plays a significant role in its pathophysiology [14]. In females, estrogens and X-inactivation can modify the immune system, potentially contributing to the higher prevalence of GD. Female tissues are mosaics, consisting of both paternal and maternal cells with an active X chromosome [15].

3. Potential factors triggering GD

There is broad agreement that identifying all potential factors involved in the pathogenesis of GD, as summarized in **Table 1**, could lead to the development of more effective treatment strategies and preventive measures [16]. This is especially critical given the current lack of an effective pharmacological therapy for GD [16–18].

Viral infection is an environmental factor associated with GD. The evidence for this link is demonstrated by the prevalence of enteroviral proteins, the upregulation of human leukocyte antigen (HLA) class I expression, and the co-localization with Stat1, VP1, and PKR, which are well-known antiviral response proteins [19].

Viral infection (SARS-CoV-2)
Pregnancy (postpartum)
Iodine excess
Emotional stress
Smoking
Helicobacter pylori infection
Alterations in gut microbiota

Table 1.
A summary of factors that may trigger the development of Graves' disease.

Recent studies suggest that SARS-CoV-2 infection may trigger GD. The growing evidence of a direct relationship between the thyroid gland and COVID-19 highlights the need for physicians to explore other potential and unknown clinical issues related to COVID-19. The angiotensin-converting enzyme 2 (ACE2) protein, which serves as the receptor for viral entry into cells, is highly expressed in thyroid tissue, as well as in other organs such as the nasopharynx and lungs. Infection in areas distant from the thyroid may also transmit the virus or activate immune cells that subsequently target the gland [20].

Several environmental factors—other than infection—including pregnancy (mainly postpartum), iodine excess, emotional stress, smoking, and interferon alpha trigger immune responses in susceptible genes to eventually cause GD [1].

In 1825, a 21-year-old woman fell from a wheelchair while descending a hill at high speed. Although she sustained minimal body injuries, the incident caused her intense fear. Following this event, she began experiencing symptoms such as nervousness, palpitations, and swelling of the thyroid gland [21]. This case is believed to be the first documented instance of new-onset thyroid disease following acute stress [22].

Measuring emotions with precision is challenging, but there has been significant progress over the past decade in improving the objectivity of methods used to quantify stressful life events [22]. In an early study of 219 individuals with GD, 95% (208 participants) reported experiencing stressful life events in the 12 months before their diagnosis. However, some studies indicate that the strength of this association may vary based on gender or age group [23].

A recent meta-analysis involving 2892 participants found that stress is a significant factor in the onset of GD [24]. The analysis revealed that the relationship between stressful life events and GD was stronger in studies with a higher proportion of female patients and weaker in studies involving older patients. These findings suggest that women may have an increased susceptibility to autoimmune thyroid disease following stressful conditions, although the exact reasons for this heightened vulnerability are not yet fully understood [22].

Studies have shown that gut microbiota are linked to autoimmune thyroid diseases [25]. Decreases in *Bifidobacterium* and *Lactobacillus* have been associated with such disorders, but microbiome data in GD are still limited [26].

The use of oral contraceptive pills appears to be protective against Graves' disease, as is male sex, suggesting that sex hormones have a significant influence on the condition [27, 28].

4. Molecular pathogenesis of GD

The development of GD starts with a failure of the immune tolerance toward the thyroid. This breakdown is mediated by a multifactorial autoimmune process in genetically predisposed subjects [7].

4.1 Autoantibodies in GD

The pathophysiological hallmark of GD is the liberation of antibodies directed against the thyroid-stimulating hormone (TSH) receptor, causing continuous thyroid stimulation and hyperthyroidism [29]. TSH receptor antibodies (TRAbs) are classified into three types: TSH receptor stimulating antibody (TSAb), TSH receptor blocking antibody (TBAb), and neutralizing antibody. Among the three subtypes, the first and second ones are clinically significant: TSAb, which stimulates the TSH receptor causing GD, and TBAb, which blocks the TSH receptor causing hypothyroidism [30].

TSAb is mainly of the IgG1 isotype. It binds to a discontinuous epitope within the leucine-rich domain of the TSH receptor's extracellular region, spanning approximately from amino acids 20 to 260 [31, 32].

TSAb—also known as thyroid-stimulating immunoglobulin (*TSI*)—is synthesized mainly by B lymphocytes present within the thyroid cells, but lymph nodes and bone marrow are other possible sites for synthesis. B lymphocytes are activated by T lymphocytes, which become sensitized after encountering an antigen in the thyroid gland [1]. TSAb exerts functional effects similar to those of TSH, as both bind to the TSH receptor on the thyroid cell membrane and activate the cyclic adenosine monophosphate (cAMP) signaling pathway. This activation leads to thyroid stimulation that occurs independently of the normal TSH feedback mechanisms (see **Figure 1**) [33, 34]. Neutralizing (apoptotic) antibodies neither stimulate nor inhibit the functional activity of the TSH receptor. However, they play a crucial role in the signaling process and can induce apoptosis in thyroid cells [33].

This B and T lymphocyte-mediated autoimmunity is directed at four known antigens in the thyroid: thyroglobulin, thyroid peroxidase, sodium-iodide symporter, and the TSH receptor. The TSH receptor represents the primary autoantigen of GD and is responsible for the manifestation of hyperthyroidism. Direct proof of an autoimmune disorder that is mediated by autoantibodies is the development of hyperthyroidism in healthy subjects by transferring TSH receptor antibodies in serum from patients with GD and the passive transfer of TSH receptor antibodies to the fetus in pregnant women [26].

The workload and personal problems may result in chronic stress that in turn induces the release of cortisol and adrenaline. This leads to the well-known stress-related health problems, including thyroid dysfunction. These stress hormones can accelerate the production of interleukins 4, 6, and 10 and inhibit the production of

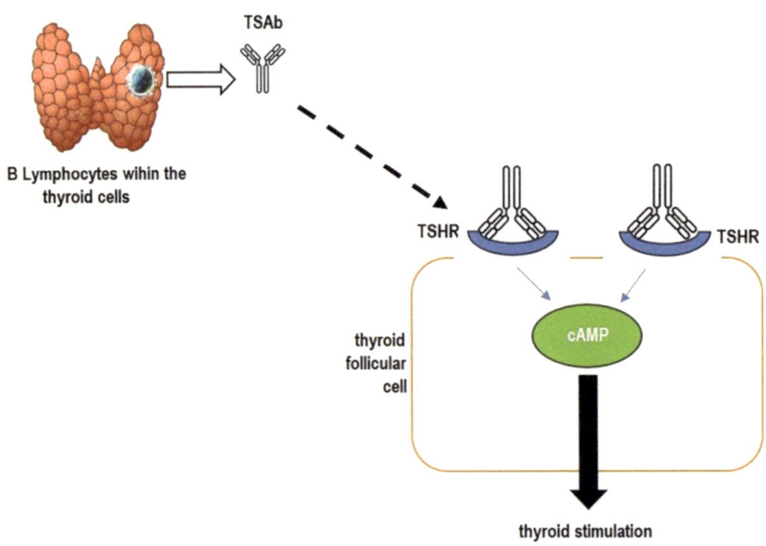

Figure 1.
Schematic representation of the mechanism of action of TSAb (TSAb = thyroid-stimulating antibody; TSHR = TSH receptor; cAMP = cyclic adenosine monophosphate).

interleukin 12 [24, 35]. They stimulate T helper (TH) 2 cells, Th17 cells, or Th1 cells and at the same time, induce apoptosis in regulatory T cells. Low levels of regulatory T cells have been noticed in patients with untreated GD, and this is inversely correlated with the serum concentration of TRAbs [22].

4.2 Cytokines in GD

Chemokines (chemotactic cytokines) are small cytokines that trigger directed chemotaxis in the neighboring responsive cells. The main subtypes of chemokines include CXC, CC, CX3C, and XC. The chemokine receptor (CXCR)3 binds CXCL11, CXCL10, and CXCL9 (that are interferon (IFN)-gamma dependent chemokine, Th1 chemokines) [36].

Early in the course of GD, CXCR3-expressing Th1 cells are programmed for the production of CXCL10 by resident epithelial cells of the thyroid follicles; this results in upcoming amplification of inflammation [37]. GD patients were shown to have levels of serum CXCL10 higher than controls matched by age and sex [38].

Circulating CXCL10 levels were similar in untreated patients in relapse of hyperthyroidism [earlier administered with Methimazole], and in untreated hyperthyroid GD patients of recent diagnosis. This indicates that active phases of the disease are associated with high serum CXCL10 in relapsing and newly diagnosed GD patients [39].

4.3 Molecular mimicry in GD

Molecular mimicry is a key mechanism through which infectious or chemical agents can trigger autoimmunity. This process occurs when similarities between foreign and self-peptides lead to the activation of autoreactive T or B cells by a foreign-derived antigen in a genetically susceptible individual [40].

Helicobacter pylori is a flagellated, microaerophilic, gram-negative bacillus [41]. Although its prevalence has decreased in developed countries, the infection remains widespread globally [42]. It has been linked to peptic ulcers and gastric cancer [43], but over the past two decades, it has also been associated with various non-gastric conditions [44], including autoimmune thyroid diseases, particularly GD [45]. The association between thyroid autoimmunity and *H. pylori* can be explained mostly by molecular mimicry [46].

H. pylori stimulates the proliferation of CD4+ lymphocytes that recognize *H. pylori* epitopes structurally similar to H/K/ATPase on stomach parietal cells. This activation leads Th1 autoreactive lymphocytes to target H/K/ATPase. Since H/K/ATPase is also present in the thyroid gland, these Th1 autoreactive lymphocytes can induce apoptosis in thyroid cells and synthesize proinflammatory cytokines, such as TNF-alpha and INF-gamma [47, 48].

5. Molecular pathogenesis of the extra-thyroidal manifestations of GD

5.1 Graves' ophthalmopathy

Graves' ophthalmopathy (GO), also known as thyroid-associated ophthalmopathy, is a vision-threatening and cosmetically damaging organ-specific autoimmune disease. It occurs in approximately 30–50% of GD patients [49]. Signs and symptoms of GO include retraction of the eyelid, proptosis, diplopia, exposure keratitis, corneal clouding and ulceration, and, in severe cases, vision-threatening compressive optic neuropathy [50].

The orbital tissues and extraocular muscles of patients with GO have extensive localized and diffuse monocyte infiltrates, along with mucopolysaccharide deposits. The infiltrating cells are predominantly CD4+ T lymphocytes, with smaller numbers of neutrophils and plasma cells present as well [50]. This suggests that the primary pathophysiology of GO is driven by cellular immunity [51].

The orbital fibroblasts (OFs) located between the extraocular muscles and infiltrating autoreactive T cells are the target cells involved in the autoimmune process of GO. T lymphocytes interact with OFs through the CD40-CD154 costimulatory pathway [50]. Activation of OFs results in the release of considerable amounts of cytokines and extracellular matrix (ECM), leading to severe orbital inflammation and tissue remodeling [51]. CD90 is a marker that can be expressed on the surface of OFs, where $CD90^{+}$ OFs are associated with fibrosis, while $CD90^{-}$ OFs are more likely to lead to adipogenesis [52]. During the active phase of orbital tissue changes, the volume of tissue around the eye increases due to inflammatory cell infiltration and orbital tissue edema, resulting in elevated intraocular pressure [53]. This causes the eye to move beyond the bony rim of the orbit, leading to exophthalmos. The major pathological changes in GO include cytokine production and inflammation, adipogenesis, hyaluronan synthesis, and myofibrillogenesis [53].

In orbital tissues, TSH receptor is also detectable, but its pathogenetic role in GO is still unclear. Overexpression of the insulin-like growth factor-1 (IGF1) receptor in orbital fibroblasts, B cells, and T cells of patients with Graves' ophthalmopathy has been documented. These patients have circulating immunoglobulins that result in increased synthesis of hyaluronan and cytokine release by binding to IGF1 receptors. These findings encouraged researchers to try using monoclonal antibodies to block IGF1 receptors, and this can reduce the expression levels of TSH receptor and IGF1 receptors on fibrocytes and antagonize TSH-induced expression of inflammation genes (IL6, IL8, and TNFA) [26].

5.2 Pretibial myxedema

Pretibial myxedema (PTM), also known as thyroid dermopathy, represents the third element in the classic triad of GD (goiter, ophthalmopathy, and pretibial myxedema). Although commonly associated with the pretibial area, this condition can also affect the ankles, dorsum of the feet, and occasionally appears on the elbows, knees, upper back, and neck [54]. It is a rare and late-stage clinical manifestation of GD, occurring in 0.5–4.3% of cases. However, in patients with GO, the prevalence can rise to 15% [55].

Patients with mild PTM are often asymptomatic, while severe cases can lead to functional difficulties, such as problems with dressing and wearing socks or shoes. Only a small number of patients may experience pain, itching, or hyperpigmentation [56, 57]. In rare instances, PTM has been associated with entrapment neuropathy and even foot drop [58]. Interestingly, PTM can sometimes be mistaken for a venous leg ulcer due to their similar clinical presentations, leading to under-recognition of the condition [59].

The exact pathogenesis of this condition remains unclear. However, it is widely regarded as an autoimmune reaction, primarily driven by autoantibodies [56, 60].

High levels of TRAbs have been observed in patients with PTM. It is believed that these antibodies target the thyrotropin receptors located in skin lesions, leading to autoimmune damage. When stimulated by the activation of humoral and cellular immune responses, fibroblasts produce large amounts of glycosaminoglycans that accumulate in the dermis and subcutaneous tissue, resulting in the development of localized myxedema [61–63].

The characteristic pathological changes in PTM include mucinous edema and the fragmentation of collagen fibers, accompanied by the deposition of acid mucopolysaccharides, particularly hyaluronic acid, in the papillary and reticular dermis. This process often extends into deeper tissues [54, 64]. Additionally, an increased number of fibroblasts have been observed in affected areas [64]. Clinically, these changes manifest as non-pitting edema of the dermis, which results from the hydrophilic nature of these substances and the secondary compression of dermal lymphatics, as well as the fragmentation of dermal collagen fibers [65].

5.3 Thyroid acropachy

Although related to thyroid dermopathy, thyroid acropachy (TAC) is a distinct and exceedingly rare manifestation (less than 1%) of GD. It is characterized by a combination of digital swelling and nail clubbing, typically associated with thyroid ophthalmopathy and dermopathy [66]. It can occur in patients who are biochemically euthyroid or hypothyroid, often following the treatment of thyrotoxicosis [56, 67]. TAC is generally considered the final manifestation after thyroid ophthalmopathy and dermopathy [68]. **Table 2** summarizes the differences between finger clubbing and TAC.

The exact pathogenesis of TAC remains unknown, but it is believed to result from stimulating autoantibodies targeting TSH and IGF1 receptors [69]. In patients with combined GO, PTM, and TAC, levels of TRAbs, TSAbs, and TBAbs are typically extremely elevated [70, 71]. It seems that TRAb molecules bind to the TSH receptors on fibroblasts in the periosteum, triggering an inflammatory response that leads to cell proliferation and glycosaminoglycan deposition [66]. The musculoskeletal manifestations of this process almost never occur without the other components of the triad—ophthalmopathy, dermopathy, and acropachy [72, 73]. Some studies also suggest that smoking may be a predisposing factor for acropachy in patients with GD [72].

	Thyroid acropachy	**Finger clubbing**
Incidence	A very rare manifestation of GD	Primary clubbing occurs in 89% of patients diagnosed with pachydermoperiostosis
Pain	Rare	Frequent
Other signs	GO and PTM	Depends upon the involved system
TRAbs	High titer	None
Spontaneous remission	Has been reported	Infrequent

Table 2.
The difference between thyroid acropachy and finger clubbing (GD: Graves' disease; GO: Graves' ophthalmopathy; PTM: pretibial myxedema).

6. Conclusion

GD is an autoimmune disorder that leads to hyperthyroidism. Factors that may trigger this disease include stress, viral infection, pregnancy, high iodine intake, and cigarette smoking. The primary feature of GD is the production of autoantibodies, particularly TSI, against TSH receptors on the thyroid gland cells. TSI mimics the action of TSH but is much more potent and persistent. Chemotactic cytokines play a role in the pathogenesis of GD, as these patients have higher serum CXCL10 levels than controls.

Conflict of interest

The author declares no conflict of interest.

Author details

Hosam Mohamad Hamza
Faculty of Medicine, Department of General Surgery, Minia University, Minia, Egypt

*Address all correspondence to: hossam.hamza@mu.edu.eg

References

[1] Pokhrel B, Bhusal K. Grave's disease. In: StatPearls. Treasure Island (FL): StatPearls Publishing; 2024. Available from: https://www.ncbi.nlm.nih.gov/books/NBK448195/. [Updated 2023 Jun 20]

[2] Hussain YS, Hookham JC, Allahabadia A, Balasubramanian SP. Epidemiology, management and outcomes of Graves' disease-real life data. Endocrine. 2017;**56**(3):568-578

[3] Prabhakar BS, Bahn RS, Smith TJ. Current perspective on the pathogenesis of Graves' disease and ophthalmopathy. Endocrine Reviews. 2003;**24**(6):802-835

[4] Brix TH, Hegedüs L. Twins as a tool for evaluating the influence of genetic susceptibility in thyroid autoimmunity. Annales d'Endocrinologie. 2011;**72**(2):103-107

[5] Brix TH, Hegedüs L. Twin studies as a model for exploring the aetiology of autoimmune thyroid disease. Clinical Endocrinology. 2012;**76**(4):457-464

[6] McLeod DS, Cooper DS, Ladenson PW, Whiteman DC, Jordan SJ. Race/ethnicity and the prevalence of thyrotoxicosis in young Americans. Thyroid. 2015;**25**(6):621-628

[7] Wémeau JL, Klein M, Sadoul JL, Briet C, Vélayoudom-Céphise FL. Graves' disease: Introduction, epidemiology, endogenous and environmental pathogenic factors. Annales d'Endocrinologie. 2018;**79**(6):599-607

[8] Chu X, Pan CM, Zhao SX, et al. A genome-wide association study identifies two new risk loci for Graves' disease. Nature Genetics. 2011;**43**(9):897-901

[9] Jacobson E, Tomer Y. The CD40, CTLA-4, thyroglobulin, TSH receptor, and PTPN22 gene quintet and its contribution to thyroid autoimmunity: Back to the future. Journal of Autoimmunity. 2007;**28**(2-3):85-98

[10] Tan G, Wang X, Zheng G, et al. Meta-analysis reveals significant association between FOXP3 polymorphisms and susceptibility to Graves' disease. The Journal of International Medical Research. 2021;**49**(4):3000605211004199

[11] Zhou F, Liang Z, Wang X, et al. The VDR gene confers a genetic predisposition to Graves' disease and Graves' ophthalmopathy in the Southwest Chinese Han population. Gene. 2021;**793**:145750

[12] Rapoport B, McLachlan SM. Graves' hyperthyroidism is antibody-mediated but is predominantly a Th1-type cytokine disease. The Journal of Clinical Endocrinology and Metabolism. 2014;**99**(11):4060-4061

[13] Rapoport B, McLachlan SM. Reflections on thyroid autoimmunity: A personal overview from the past into the future. Hormone and Metabolic Research. 2018;**50**(12):840-852

[14] Antonelli A, Ferrari SM, Ragusa F, Elia G, Paparo SR, Ruffilli I, et al. Graves' disease: Epidemiology, genetic and environmental risk factors and viruses. Best Practice & Research. Clinical Endocrinology & Metabolism. 2020;**34**(1):101387

[15] Brooks WH. X chromosome inactivation and autoimmunity. Clinical Reviews in Allergy and Immunology. 2010;**39**(1):20-29

[16] Tanda ML, Piantanida E, Lai A, et al. Thyroid autoimmunity and environment.

Hormone and Metabolic Research. 2009;**41**(6):436-442

[17] Masiello E, Veronesi G, Gallo D, et al. Antithyroid drug treatment for Graves' disease: Baseline predictive models of relapse after treatment for a patient-tailored management. Journal of Endocrinological Investigation. 2018;**41**(12):1425-1432

[18] Bartalena L, Piantanida E, Tanda ML. Can a patient-tailored treatment approach for Graves' disease reduce mortality? The Lancet Diabetes and Endocrinology. 2019;**7**(4):245-246

[19] Weider T, Richardson S, Morgan N, et al. HLA class I upregulation and antiviral immune responses in Graves' disease. The Journal of Clinical Endocrinology and Metabolism. 2021;**106**(4):e1763-e1774

[20] Murugan A, Alzahrani A. SARS-CoV-2 plays a pivotal role in inducing hyperthyroidism of Graves' disease. Endocrine. 2021;**73**(2):243-254

[21] Graves RJ. Newly observed affection of the thyroid gland in females. Clinical lectures. London Medical and Surgical Journal. 1835;**7**:516-517

[22] Noreña J, Desai K. Managing Stress for a Healthier Thyroid. Medscape; 2024. Available from: https://www.medscape.com/viewarticle/1000132

[23] Winsa B, Adami H, Bergström R, et al. Stressful life events and Graves' disease. Lancet. 1991;**338**(8781):1475-1479

[24] Wang J, Chen Z, Carru C, et al. What is the impact of stress on the onset and anti-thyroid drug therapy in patients with graves' disease: A systematic review and meta-analysis. BMC Endocrine Disorders. 2023;**23**(1):194

[25] Gong B, Wang C, Meng F, et al. Association between gut microbiota and autoimmune thyroid disease: A systematic review and meta-analysis. Frontiers in Endocrinology (Lausanne). 2021;**12**:774362

[26] Yeung S, Habra M, Chiu A, Khardori R. Graves Disease. Medscape Endocrinology. Available from: https://emedicine.medscape.com/article/120619-overview. [updated 2023 Jan 4]

[27] Smith TJ, Hegedüs L. Graves' disease. The New England Journal of Medicine. 2016;**375**(16):1552-1565

[28] Strieder TG, Prummel MF, Tijssen JG, Endert E, Wiersinga WM. Risk factors for and prevalence of thyroid disorders in a cross-sectional study among healthy female relatives of patients with autoimmune thyroid disease. Clinical Endocrinology. 2003;**59**(3):396-401

[29] Alvin Mathew A, Papaly R, Maliakal A, Chandra L, Antony MA. Elevated Graves' disease-specific thyroid-stimulating immunoglobulin and thyroid stimulating hormone receptor antibody in a patient with subacute thyroiditis. Cureus. 2021;**13**(11):e19448

[30] Takasu N, Oshiro C, Akamine H, et al. Thyroid-stimulating antibody and TSH-binding inhibitor immunoglobulin in 277 Graves' patients and in 686 normal subjects. Journal of Endocrinological Investigation. 1997;**20**(8):452-461

[31] Rapoport B, Chazenbalk GD, Jaume JC, McLachlan SM. The thyrotropin (TSH) receptor: Interaction with TSH and autoantibodies. Endocrine Reviews. 1998;**19**(6):673-716

[32] Rapoport B, McLachlan SM. TSH receptor cleavage into subunits and

shedding of the A-subunit; A molecular and clinical perspective. Endocrine Reviews. 2016;**37**(2):114-134

[33] Gao Y, Qiu L, Yu S, Cheng X. Thyroid stimulating receptor autoantibodies. Clinica Chimica Acta. 2024;**559**:119700

[34] Diana T, Olivo PD, Chang YH, et al. Comparison of a novel homogeneous cyclic amp assay and a luciferase assay for measuring stimulating thyrotropin-receptor autoantibodies. European Thyroid Journal. 2020;**9**(2):67-72

[35] Falgarone G, Heshmati HM, Cohen R, Reach G. Mechanisms in endocrinology. Role of emotional stress in the pathophysiology of Graves' disease. European Journal of Endocrinology. 2012;**168**(1):R13-R18

[36] Lasagni L, Francalanci M, Annunziato F, et al. An alternatively spliced variant of CXCR3 mediates the inhibition of endothelial cell growth induced by IP-10, Mig, and I-TAC, and acts as functional receptor for platelet factor 4. The Journal of Experimental Medicine. 2003;**197**(11):1537-1549

[37] Romagnani P, Rotondi M, Lazzeri E, et al. Expression of IP-10/CXCL10 and MIG/CXCL9 in the thyroid and increased levels of IP-10/CXCL10 in the serum of patients with recent-onset Graves' disease. The American Journal of Pathology. 2002;**161**(1):195-206

[38] Antonelli A, Rotondi M, Ferrari SM, et al. Interferon-gamma-inducible alpha-chemokine CXCL10 involvement in Graves' ophthalmopathy: Modulation by peroxisome proliferator-activated receptor-gamma agonists. The Journal of Clinical Endocrinology and Metabolism. 2006;**91**(2):614-620

[39] Antonelli A, Rotondi M, Fallahi P, et al. Increase of interferon-gamma-inducible CXC chemokine CXCL10 serum levels in patients with active Graves' disease, and modulation by methimazole therapy. Clinical Endocrinology. 2006;**64**(2):189-195

[40] Rojas M, Restrepo-Jiménez P, Monsalve DM, et al. Molecular mimicry and autoimmunity. Journal of Autoimmunity. 2018;**95**:100-123

[41] Gu H. Role of flagella in the pathogenesis of *Helicobacter pylori*. Current Microbiology. 2017;**74**(7):863-869

[42] Mentis A, Lehours P, Mégraud F. Epidemiology and diagnosis of *Helicobacter pylori* infection. Helicobacter. 2015;**20**(Suppl 1):1-7

[43] Burucoa C, Axon A. Epidemiology of *Helicobacter pylori* infection. Helicobacter. 2017;**22**(Suppl):1

[44] de Korwin JD, Ianiro G, Gibiino G, Gasbarrini A. *Helicobacter pylori* infection and extragastric diseases in 2017. Helicobacter. 2017;**22**(Suppl):1

[45] Smyk DS, Koutsoumpas AL, Mytilinaiou MG, Rigopoulou EI, Sakkas LI, Bogdanos DP. *Helicobacter pylori* and autoimmune disease: Cause or bystander. World Journal of Gastroenterology. 2014;**20**(3):613-629

[46] Cuan-Baltazar Y, Soto-Vega E. Microorganisms associated to thyroid autoimmunity. Autoimmunity Reviews. 2020;**19**(9):102614

[47] Choi YM, Kim TY, Kim EY, et al. Association between thyroid autoimmunity and *Helicobacter pylori* infection. The Korean Journal of Internal Medicine. 2017;**32**(2):309-313

[48] Wang L, Cao ZM, Zhang LL, et al. *Helicobacter pylori* and autoimmune

diseases: Involving multiple systems. Frontiers in Immunology. 2022;**13**:833424

[49] Elia G, Fallahi P, Ragusa F, Paparo SR, Mazzi V, Benvenga S, et al. Precision medicine in Graves' disease and ophthalmopathy. Frontiers in Pharmacology. 2021;**12**:754386. DOI: 10.3389/fphar.2021.754386

[50] Bahn RS. Graves' ophthalmopathy. The New England Journal of Medicine. 2010;**362**(8):726-738

[51] Zheng J, Duan H, You S, et al. Research progress on the pathogenesis of Graves' ophthalmopathy: Based on immunity, noncoding RNA and exosomes. Frontiers in Immunology. 2022;**13**:952954

[52] Fang S, Huang Y, Zhong S, et al. Regulation of orbital fibrosis and adipogenesis by pathogenic Th17 cells in Graves orbitopathy. The Journal of Clinical Endocrinology and Metabolism. 2017;**102**(11):4273-4283

[53] Łacheta D, Miśkiewicz P, Głuszko A, Nowicka G, Struga M, Kantor I, et al. Immunological aspects of Graves' ophthalmopathy. BioMed Research International. 2019;**2019**:7453260

[54] Doshi DN, Blyumin ML, Kimball AB. Cutaneous manifestations of thyroid disease. Clinics in Dermatology. 2008;**26**(3):283-287

[55] Schwartz KM, Fatourechi V, Ahmed DD, Pond GR. Dermopathy of Graves' disease (pretibial myxedema): Long-term outcome. The Journal of Clinical Endocrinology and Metabolism. 2002;**87**(2):438-446

[56] Bartalena L, Fatourechi V. Extrathyroidal manifestations of Graves' disease: A 2014 update. Journal of Endocrinological Investigation. 2014;**37**(8):691-700

[57] Lohiya S, Lohiya V, Stahl EJ. Pretibial myxedema without ophthalmopathy: An initial presentation of Graves' disease. The American Journal of the Medical Sciences. 2013;**346**(1):73-75

[58] Siegler M, Refetoff S. Pretibial myxedema—A reversible cause of foot drop due to entrapment of the peroneal nerve. The New England Journal of Medicine. 1976;**294**(25):1383-1384

[59] Herskovitz I, Hughes O, MacQuhae F, Kirsner RS. Pretibial myxedema masquerading as a venous leg ulcer. Wounds. 2017;**29**(3):77-79

[60] Kim WB, Mistry N, Alavi A, Sibbald C, Sibbald RG. Pretibial myxedema: Case presentation and review of treatment options. The International Journal of Lower Extremity Wounds. 2014;**13**(2):152-154

[61] Takasu N, Higa H, Kinjou Y. Treatment of pretibial myxedema (PTM) with topical steroid ointment application with sealing cover (steroid occlusive dressing technique: Steroid ODT) in Graves' patients. Internal Medicine. 2010;**49**(7):665-669

[62] Deng A, Song D. Multipoint subcutaneous injection of long-acting glucocorticid as a cure for pretibial myxedema. Thyroid. 2011;**21**(1):83-85

[63] Kamath C, Young S, Kabelis K, et al. Thyrotrophin receptor antibody characteristics in a woman with long-standing Hashimoto's who developed Graves' disease and pretibial myxoedema. Clinical Endocrinology. 2012;**77**(3):465-470

[64] Shishido M, Kuroda K, Tsukifuji R, et al. A case of pretibial myxedema

associated with Graves' disease: An immunohistochemical study of serum-derived hyaluronan-associated protein. The Journal of Dermatology. 1995;**22**(12):948-952

[65] Bull RH, Coburn PR, Mortimer PS. Pretibial myxoedema: A manifestation of lymphoedema? Lancet. 1993;**341**(8842):403-404

[66] Fatourechi V, Ahmed DD, Schwartz KM. Thyroid acropachy: Report of 40 patients treated at a single institution in a 26-year period. The Journal of Clinical Endocrinology and Metabolism. 2002;**87**(12):5435-5441

[67] Scanlon GT, Clemett AR. Thyroid acropachy. Radiology. 1964;**83**:1039-1042

[68] Cohen B, Cadesky A, Jaggi S. Dermatologic manifestations of thyroid disease: A literature review. Frontiers in Endocrinology (Lausanne). 2023;**14**:1167890. DOI: 10.3389/fendo.2023.1167890

[69] Jadidi J, Sigari M, Efendizade A, et al. Thyroid acropachy: A rare skeletal manifestation of autoimmune thyroid disease. Radiology Case Reports. 2019;**14**(8):917-919

[70] Taguchi T, Nakajima H, Terada Y. Graves' dermopathy and acropachy. Endocrine. 2015;**49**(1):296-297

[71] Elsayad K, Kriz J, Bauch J, et al. Radiation therapy as part of the therapeutic regimen for extensive multilocular myxedema in a patient with exophthalmos, myxedema and osteoarthropathy syndrome: A case report. Oncology Letters. 2015;**9**(5):2404-2408

[72] Anwar S, Gibofsky A. Musculoskeletal manifestations of thyroid disease. Rheumatic Diseases Clinics of North America. 2010;**36**(4):637-646

[73] Boswell SB, Patel DB, White EA, et al. Musculoskeletal manifestations of endocrine disorders. Clinical Imaging. 2014;**38**(4):384-396

Section 2

Graves' Disease Diagnostic Aspects

Chapter 3

Graves' Disease: Novel Diagnostic Approaches and Emerging Treatment Options

Ruchi Agrawal and Shahnaz Ahmad

Abstract

The fundamental pathophysiology of Graves' hyperthyroidism involves the activation of the thyroid-stimulating hormone receptor [TSHR] by autoantibodies, resulting in excessive thyroid hormone secretion independent of the hypothalamic-pituitary-thyroid [HPT] axis and consequently leading to the clinical symptoms and signs of hyperthyroidism. Graves' hyperthyroidism has been linked with significant morbidity and reduced quality of life. Over the past 70 years, the treatment options for Graves' hyperthyroidism have remained unchanged and include antithyroid medications, radioiodine ablation, and surgery. Antithyroid drugs [ATDs] lack long-term efficacy, while treatment with radioiodine therapy and surgical intervention is associated with increased morbidity and a lifelong need for thyroxine replacement. Moreover, no treatments have been developed to target the fundamental immunopathogenesis of the disease until now. The increasing need for effective treatments has driven the investigation of novel therapeutic strategies for Graves' hyperthyroidism. Current therapies under investigation include biologics, small molecules, peptide immunomodulation, and TSHR-specific treatment modalities. These emerging therapies offer new hope in the management of Graves' hyperthyroidism, potentially surpassing the currently available treatments. In the near future, these therapies may become the first line of management. This chapter explores the diagnostic and therapeutic advancements in Graves' hyperthyroidism.

Keywords: Graves' disease, TSH receptor, rituximab, BAFF, TSH specific immunotherapy

1. Introduction

Graves' disease is a multisystem autoimmune disorder characterized by the production of autoantibodies targeting the TSH receptor. These autoantibodies bind to and activate the TSH receptor, and the resultant hyperstimulation of the thyroid gland induces excessive thyroid hormone synthesis and secretion. The autoimmune nature of this disorder arises from a complex interplay of genetic predispositions and environmental influences [1, 2].

2. Epidemiology

The predominant hyperthyroidism is Graves" disease worldwide, with an annual incidence of 20 to 50 cases per 100,000 [3]. The age incidence of the disease shows predominant peak at 30–50 years of age, although no age group is entirely exempt. Women face a 3% lifetime risk compared to 0.5% for men. While long-term changes in iodine intake do not influence the risk, a sudden increase in iodine intake can temporarily elevate the incidence. The annual incidence of Graves" disease-related eye complications is 16 cases per 100,000 women and 3 cases per 100,000 men. The condition is more prevalent in the white population compared to Asians [4]. Severe eye complications are more likely to develop in older men than in younger individuals [5].

3. Pathogenesis

The precise etiology of Graves" disease remains elusive. The interplay between genetic and epigenetic elements is believed to underlie the pathogenesis of Graves" disease. Genome-wide association studies have identified numerous genetic loci conferring susceptibility to Graves" disease [1, 2, 6]. Genetic susceptibility to autoimmune diseases has been linked to genes involved in thyroid function and immune regulation, including thyroglobulin, thyrotropin receptor, HLA-DRβ, PTPN22, CTLA4, CD25, and CD40 [1]. The genes responsible for thyrotropin receptors and T-cell signaling have been found to be hypermethylated, potentially disrupting normal thyroid function [6]. Environmental factors such as dietary iodine intake, tobacco smoke exposure, infections, and emotional stress are often implicated in the disease's onset. Administration of Alemtuzumab, a monoclonal antibody directed against CD52, has been associated with increased incidence of Graves" disease [7]. The complex mechanism by which these factors influence disease susceptibility is still unclear [8].

3.1 Anti-thyrotropin receptor antibody

IgG1 antibodies are usually produced early in the immunogenicity and are mainly induced by TH1 cells. IgG4 antibodies are characteristically induced after prolonged antigen stimulation and are predominantly facilitated with the help of TH2 cells. In Graves' disease, the antibodies that activate thyrotropin receptors in the thyroid gland are of the IgG1 subclass. In both Graves' disease and Hashimoto thyroiditis, TPO Ab and Tg Ab can belong to either IgG1 or IgG4 subclass. This concludes that Graves' disease is characterized by dual involvement of TH1 and TH2 cells [9]. Autoantibodies play a crucial role in causing Graves' disease, and their production is supported by the specific focus nature of immune response, that is, oligoclonality and light chain restriction [10, 11]. These autoantibodies cause the thyroid to produce hormones in an uncontrolled manner, bypassing regulation by the hypothalamic-pituitary axis. The activating antibodies mimic the function of thyrotropin at its receptor, triggering a similar but distinct signaling pathway [12]. In addition to activating antibodies, there can be blocking antibodies, which result in hypothyroidism. The balance between the stimulatory and blocking antibodies determines the level of thyroid function. These antibodies recognize a specific part called as epitope on the alpha subunit of the TSH receptor. Recent studies have found that the multimedia form of this alpha subunit is important in the affinity maturation of these antibodies [13]. Besides stimulatory antibodies, patients with Graves" disease have antibodies against thyroglobulin (Tg) and antithyroid peroxidase (anti-TPO), which are non-pathogenic. Antibodies against IGF-1 receptors have been identified in patients with Graves' disease, suggesting a role in the pathogenesis of Graves' orbitopathy [14].

3.2 The adaptive immune response in Graves" disease

B and T lymphocytes, which are critical components of the adaptive immune system, are essential contributors to the development of Graves" disease. Thyroid autoimmunity results from the breakdown of self-tolerance. There are two forms of self-tolerance: central and peripheral. Central tolerance occurs in the thymus and bone marrow, where self-reactive T and B cells are eliminated during their development. Peripheral tolerance encompasses mechanisms that regulate self-reactive cells that have evaded central tolerance, preventing them from initiating an autoimmune response. The failure of these tolerance mechanisms leads to the production of autoantibodies and the autoimmune response characteristic of Graves" disease [15]. During the process of development, the immature T cells enter the thymus, where a critical process of positive selection occurs. Immature T cells interact with the self-peptides presented by the thymic epithelial cells. T cells that do not recognize self-peptides [no affinity] or recognize them with very strongly [high affinity] undergo apoptosis [a process of negative selection]. The T cells that recognize self-peptides with moderate affinity are positively selected to mature and leave the thymus as functional T cells. Thus, the immune system ensures that it is active against pathogens and tolerant to self-antigens [16]. TSH receptor gene is normally expressed in the thyroid gland where its expression will help regulate thyroid function. However, in people with Graves" disease, the full-length TSH receptor gene can also be found in higher amounts in hyperplastic thymus [17]. Genetic epigenetic interactions involving a non-coding single nucleotide polymorphism [SNP] in the TSH receptor gene regulate the TSH receptor gene expression. This may facilitate the escape of TSH receptor reactive T cells from central tolerance in the thymus, thereby triggering Graves" disease [18]. Central tolerance sometimes fails to eliminate all self-reactive T cells. In such cases, peripheral tolerance comes into play. Peripheral tolerance controls autoreactive T cells through the engagement of cytotoxic T-lymphocyte-associated protein [CTLA-4], resulting in T cell anergy. T regulatory cells are generated in the thymus in response to self-antigen presentation. These natural T regulatory cells inhibit self-reactive T cells in peripheral tissues that have escaped central tolerance. Additionally, inducible T regulatory cells are generated in the periphery in response to antigen stimulation. T regulatory cells have specific surface markers, including CD4, CD25 [the IL-2 receptor alpha chain important for responding to IL-2], and FOXP3 [a transcription factor that regulates the activity of genes involved in T regulatory function]. These markers enable T regulatory cells to control other immune cells like CD4 and CD8 T cells. They also secrete cytokines such as IL-10 and TGF-beta, which suppress the immune response and inflammation. In conclusion, activation and proliferation of self-reactive T cells are prevented by T regulatory cells, thereby maintaining self-tolerance [19]. Another subset of T helper cells, known as TH17 cells, is induced by IL-6. These cells are highly proinflammatory and produce IL-17, which exacerbates autoimmune responses. For immune homeostasis, there should be a balance between TH17 cells and T regulatory cells. Studies have reported a decrease in the number of T regulatory cells and an increase in the number of TH17 cells in the peripheral blood of patients with Graves" disease. This imbalance is associated with the presence of stimulating TSH receptor antibodies and shows improvement upon methimazole treatment [16, 20–22]. In an animal model of Graves" disease researchers have observed low levels of regulatory T cells and high levels of IL-1 [23]. B cells transform into plasma cells that produce antibodies through a two-step process. Initially, an antigen binds to the B-cell receptor. Following this, the CD40 protein on the B cell interacts with the CD40 ligand on T cells, leading to the release of signaling molecules such as interleukin-4. These signals enable B cells to produce antibodies and switch their antibody class from IgM to IgG or IgE. In the thyroid, B cells exhibit a diminished response to growth signals but continue to autonomously produce anti-thyrotropin receptor antibodies. These thyroid B cells are believed to be the primary source of these antibodies, although B cells in the bloodstream may also contribute [24].

3.3 Thyroid epithelial cells

The precise role of thyroid epithelial cells in the pathogenesis of Graves" disease remains incompletely understood. These cells express specific proteins such as the thyrotropin receptor, thyroglobulin, and thyroperoxidase, which are crucial for thyroid function. The secretion of chemokine by these cells promotes the infiltration of immune cells [25]. In Graves" disease, thyroid epithelial cells begin to express MHC class II molecules, likely influenced by interferon-γ produced by infiltrating lymphocytes [26]. Although not professional antigen-presenting cells, thyroid epithelial cells can potentially present thyroid antigens to T cells. Furthermore, their expression of CD40 suggests they can directly engage with antigen-specific T cells in Graves" disease [27]. In tandem, this information suggests that thyroid epithelial cells play a passive, secondary role in the immunopathogenesis of Graves" disease, becoming more involved after immune cells have infiltrated the thyroid tissue [28].

3.4 The TSH receptor, the major autoantigen in Graves" disease

The TSHR gene is located on chromosome 14q13. It encodes a receptor known as the TSHR, which belongs to the family of G-protein-coupled receptors. This receptor has seven transmembrane segments: a large part that faces outside the cell and a smaller part that faces inside the cell. In studies involving mice, researchers induced Graves" hyperthyroidism by genetically stimulating the production of antibodies against TSHR [TSHRAb], resulting in hyperthyroidism. The TSH holoreceptor is a glycosylated protein weighing approximately 100 kDa, consisting of 744 amino acids and a single 20 amino acid peptide. It is split into two subunits, alpha and beta, connected by a disulfide bond. The alpha subunit, which is water soluble and heavily glycosylated, weighs around 50 kDa. The beta subunit, weighing about 30 kDa, is water-insoluble and contains membrane-spanning domains with three loops facing outside the cell and three loops facing inside. It shares about 70–75% similarity with the LH/hCG receptor. Both TSH and TSHRAb bind to the leucine-rich repeat region found on the alpha subunit of the TSH holoreceptor. The holoreceptor's hinge region experiences cleavage caused by disulfide bond breakage. This process leads to the shedding of the α-subunit from the receptor's extracellular side. In Graves" disease, it appears that the shed α-subunit, rather than the intact holoreceptor, acts as the autoantigen [29]. The increase in serum TSHRAb concentrations following radioiodine therapy may be due to enhanced release of the α-subunit from damaged follicular cells [30]. Stimulating TSHRAbs, extracted from individuals with Graves"

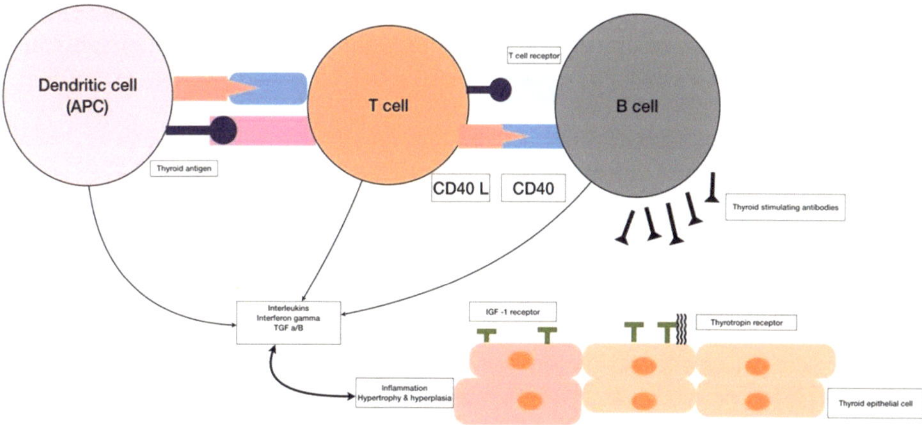

Figure 1.
Development of Graves" disease: Thyroid-stimulating hormone receptor antibody [TRAb] will stimulate thyroid cells to release T3 and T4, leading to symptoms and signs of Graves" disease. B cells regulated by T cells produce these antibodies. This process is facilitated by insulin-like growth factor (IGF-1) secreted by the liver. Antigen-presenting cells, which may include thyroid cells, B, macrophages or dendritic cells, present TSH receptor peptide to the T cells, which then get activated.

hyperthyroidism, bind to the TSHR and activate the Gαs and Gq signaling cascades, resulting in thyroid hypertrophy, augmented vascularization, and elevated synthesis and release of thyroid hormones [31, 32]. Conversely, certain TSHRAbs function as TSH antagonists, known as blocking TSHRAbs; these may be observed in some cases of autoimmune hypothyroidism and following treatment of Graves" hyperthyroidism. Neutral or cleavage-region TSHRAbs neither inhibit TSH binding nor impede TSH action; they fail to induce cAMP but possess the capacity to trigger apoptosis by targeting the hinge region (**Figure 1**) [31].

4. Pathology

In Graves" hyperthyroidism, the thyroid gland typically exhibits diffuse enlargement and uniform involvement, often referred to as diffuse toxic goiter [33]. It is exceedingly rare for the disease to be confined to a single lobe, which complicates understanding unilateral Graves' hyperthyroidism, given the systemic presence of thyroid-stimulating immunoglobulins [TSIs] [34].

Histologically, follicles in Graves' hyperthyroidism appear small and are lined with hyperplastic columnar epithelium. These follicles contain minimal colloid with noticeable marginal scalloping and vacuolization. Papillary projections from the hyperplastic epithelium extend into the follicular lumina, and there is increased vascularity. Lymphocytes and plasma cells infiltrate variably, forming aggregates that occasionally develop B-cell germinal centres, in contrast to the abundant presence seen in Hashimoto's disease. In affected areas, thyroid epithelial cells express human leukocyte antigen [HLA] class II antigens, a feature absent in normal thyroid glands. These epithelial cells may enlarge, possibly due to local stimulation by TSH receptor antibodies [TSHRAbs]. The intrathyroidal lymphocytic population is diverse, comprising mainly B cells, T helper 1 [Th1], and Th2 lymphocytes, with fewer Th17 and regulatory T cells. Treatment with iodine or antithyroid drugs [ATDs] can lead to thyroid gland involution as TSHRAbs decrease. Consequently, hyperplasia and vascularity diminish, papillary projections recede, and follicles enlarge, once again becoming filled with colloid [33].

5. Diagnosis of Graves' disease

Hyperthyroidism can result from various causes of toxicosis, with Graves' disease being the most prevalent. Other notable causes include functioning thyroid adenoma, toxic multinodular goiter, and subacute destructive thyroiditis, often triggered by viral infections, autoimmune responses, or medication. Graves' disease, a form of thyrotoxicosis, shares many clinical signs and symptoms with other hyperthyroid conditions [35]. Graves' disease is often present with extrathyroidal manifestations in the form of thyroid ophthalmopathy [36], thyroid acropachy and thyroid dermopathy [37]. There is no doubt in the diagnosis of Graves' disease when these distinct symptoms are observed alongside hyperthyroidism and diffuse goiter. Differentiating Graves' disease from other causes of hyperthyroidism, such as toxic adenoma or toxic multinodular goiter, becomes challenging in patients without obvious hyperthyroidism or ocular signs and with nodular or absent goiter. In elderly patients, Graves' disease diagnosis can be particularly difficult, as hyperthyroidism often presents with few symptoms and signs called as apathetic hyperthyroidism [38]. Furthermore, rare occurrences have been documented of euthyroid Graves' disease, where patients exhibit Graves' ophthalmopathy without hyperthyroidism. These patients show typical clinical and radiological signs of Graves' ophthalmopathy and often develop classic Graves' disease over time [39]. A survey conducted on 542 respondents revealed that the majority of respondents would order TSH receptor antibodies in addition to thyroid-stimulating hormone and free thyroxine levels [40].

5.1 Serum measurements of TSH/T3/T4

A survey conducted by members of Endocrine Society, the American Thyroid Association [ATA], members of the Endocrine Society, the American Thyroid Association [ATA] and the American Association of Clinical Endocrinologists [AACE] revealed that 90% of the endocrinologists simultaneously request the measurement of serum TSH and free T4 levels when hyperthyroidism is suspected [41]. This is in line with ATA and AACE guidelines for the diagnosis of hyperthyroidism [42]. Increased levels of free T4, along with decreased levels of TSH, confirm the diagnosis of Graves' disease [41]. Serum T3 levels are generally not measured; only 2–4% of Graves' disease patients have normal T4 levels and increased T3 levels, known as T3 toxicosis [35]. Thus, in the initial assessment of thyroid status in a patient with suspected hyperthyroidism, all three should be measured, that is, free T3, free T4 and TSH.

5.2 Serum levels of TRAB

Graves' disease is characterized by the production of autoantibodies against thyroid antigens. These autoantibodies, particularly the TRAB antibodies, play a major role in the disease. They stimulate the thyroid gland, leading to overproduction of thyroid hormones, increased thyrocyte growth and thyroid gland enlargement. [43]. The pioneering receptor assay developed by Rees Smith and Hall (1974) led the groundwork for TRAb detection by using Graves' disease patient's thyroid tissue and bovine TSH, which is iodine 125 labeled [44]. The development of TRAb assays progressed from first-generation liquid phase assay [detergent-solubilized TSH receptors) which had low sensitivity to second-generation solid phase assay developed in 1990, it had improved sensitivity and diagnostic accuracy [45]. A significant progress in TRAb assays occurred in 2002, when Sanders et al. developed thyroid-stimulating monoclonal antibodies of human origin, specifically M22. M22 replaced the bovine TSH in competitive assays, leading to third-generation assay and improved sensitivity [46]. A multicenter study evaluated the fully automated electrochemiluminescence assay for Graves' disease, yielding sensitivity and specificity of 99%, cut-off value of 1.75 IU/L. [47]. According to a meta-analysis, statistical comparison between the second- and third-generation assay in the diagnosis of Graves' disease, revealed no significant difference, confirming equal diagnostic yield [48].

5.3 Thyroid ultrasound

Thyroid ultrasonography is a non-invasive, highly sensitive, and cost-effective radiation-free imaging method. It is particularly valuable for swiftly diagnosing both nodular thyroid disorders and Graves' disease [49].

In patients with Graves' disease, conventional gray-scale ultrasonography typically reveals a diffusely enlarged thyroid gland that appears hypoechoic. This characteristic appearance aids in the diagnosis alongside clinical findings and laboratory tests [50]. A study including 426 patients with Graves' disease found that thyroid ultrasonography had a sensitivity of 95.2% in detecting abnormalities, slightly lower than thyroid scintigraphy's sensitivity of 97.4%. However, ultrasonography significantly outperformed thyroid scintigraphy in detecting concurrent nodular lesions, identifying such lesions in 16% of patients compared to only 2% by thyroid scintigraphy [51]. Furthermore, ultrasound is considered more cost-effective than thyroid scintigraphy, making it a preferred imaging modality in clinical practice for evaluating thyroid abnormalities in Graves' disease and other thyroid disorders [51].

5.4 Color flow Doppler ultrasonography

In Graves' disease, there is normal nodule vascularity with increased extra nodular vascularity. In toxic multinodular goiter, there is increased intra-nodular and peri-nodular vascularity with normal extra-nodular vascularity [52]. Color flow Doppler also distinguishes between destructive thyroiditis and Graves' disease [53].

5.5 Radioactive uptake and thyroid scan

A radioiodine uptake test and thyroid scan provide a precise evaluation of thyroid function. A small dose of radioactive iodine [123I] is given orally, and images are captured 24 hours later to measure how much iodine the thyroid gland has absorbed. Paired with low TSH levels, elevated or normal radioiodine uptake indicates thyroid hormone synthesis, which is not dependent on TSH. Low radioiodine uptake (<1%) suggests destructive thyroiditis (release of preformed hormones), struma ovarii or factitious thyrotoxicosis. Graves' disease is diagnosed by diffuse radiotracer uptake while multinodular goiter is diagnosed by patchy uptake [52, 53].

5.6 Current treatment options and their disadvantages

There are three established methods for the treatment of Graves' disease. These are antithyroid drugs (ATD) to reduce the production of thyroid hormones, radioiodine ablation (RAI) and surgical thyroidectomy. Of all the methods available, ATD is the preferred choice by most of the patients [54]. ATDs inhibit iodination, a process catalyzed by thyroid peroxidase. Methimazole [MMI] is a well-known and widely used ATD [55]. MMI is regarded as the standard ATD due to its high efficacy, acceptable side effects, and longest half-life [56]. In contrast, carbimazole [CBM], an inactive drug that is quickly metabolized into MMI in the bloodstream, is less commonly available globally and is roughly half as potent as MMI at equivalent doses [57]. Propylthiouracil [PTU] is the least potent ATD, being ten times less potent than MMI at the same dose. However, the overall efficacy of ATD treatment remains limited. ATD treatment risks include agranulocytosis, hepatotoxicity, pancreatitis and ANCA-positive vasculitis; these all can be potentially life-threatening.

Patients who still have high TRAB levels or hyperthyroidism after 18 months of maintenance therapy, or those who experience a recurrence after finishing their MMI treatment, can opt for more definitive treatments like radioactive iodine [RAI] or total thyroidectomy [TX]. TX should be done by a skilled thyroid surgeon, while RAI should be avoided in patients with Graves' disease who have active eye disease [Graves' ophthalmopathy (GO)] or a history of smoking [58]. However, there are many disadvantages with the currently available treatment. The remission rates are 45.3% with ATD, 81.5% with radioactive iodine and 96.3% with surgery [59]. Though ATD is a preferred treatment by most people, frequent relapses are the main problem with ATD and higher recurrence is seen with large size of goiter [59]. Tools like the GREAT [Graves' Recurrent Events After Therapy] score and the Clinical Severity Score [CSS] have been developed to predict the likelihood of relapse after treatment [60]. Radioactive iodine therapy is associated with an increased risk of lifetime hypothyroidism and risk of worsening Graves' ophthalmopathy due to an increase in titres of TRAB after RAI treatment [61]. After total thyroidectomy, a patient needs lifelong LT4 replacement. Also, there is increased morbidity after surgery, inadvertent removal of parathyroid may lead to lifelong disturbed Calcium phosphorus homeostasis [62]. There is a risk of recurrent laryngeal nerve injury and increased hospital stay [63]. None of the current treatment options target the key immunopathogenic mechanism.

6. Novel therapeutic strategies for Graves' disease

With a better understanding of the immunopathogenesis of Graves' disease and the disadvantages of the currently used treatment, newer treatment regimens are in development. These are currently under investigation and may become the future treatment options for Graves' disease. These include biologics, small molecule peptides, immunomodulators and teprotumumab.

6.1 B-lymphocyte depletion [CD20 depletion]

B cells exhibit a multifunctional role in autoimmunity encompassing antibody production, antigen presentation, and modulation of T cell responses [64]. Pichurin et al. demonstrated the importance of B cells in T cell activation in Graves' disease

[65]. Rituximab is an anti-CD 20 monoclonal antibody. It has been used for more than 20 years to treat lymphoproliferative malignancies like lymphoma. Also, there is increasing use in conditions like RA, SLE and myasthenia gravis [66]. The exact mechanism of action is not fully understood; however, it appears to deplete B cells by three mechanisms. These are (1) direct apoptosis, (2) complement-mediated cytotoxicity, and (3) antibody-dependent cellular cytotoxicity [67]. CD 20 is found on the surface of B lineage lymphocytes, which include early pre-B cells, mature B cells, and memory B cells; rituximab causes rapid depletion of circulating B lymphocytes within a few hours. However, as B cells mature into antibody-secreting plasma cells, they lose CD20 protein. Plasma cells which do not express CD20 and some memory B cells in lymphoid tissue survive the action of rituximab. This allows the immune system to continue functioning, and individuals can still respond to infections and previously vaccinated pathogens [68].

Several groups have investigated the role of rituximab in Graves' hyperthyroidism. Cheetam et al. conducted a phase 2 trial in total 27 patients diagnosed with Graves' hyperthyroidism between 12 and 20 years of age. They were enrolled within 6 weeks after initiation of ATD. After a single 500 mg IV dose of rituximab, the ATD was titrated and stopped at 12 months. The proportion of patients in remission at 24 months was 48%. There were no serious adverse effects and rituximab was well tolerated [69]. A study conducted by Fassi et al. demonstrated that combination of rituximab and methimazole resulted in prolonged remission in patients with Graves' disease, although TRAb antibody titer remained unaffected. There was marked reduction in stimulatory capacity of TRAb antibody on treatment with rituximab and methimazole as compared to methimazole therapy alone [70]. Heemstra et al. conducted another small prospective study involving 13 patients with recurrent Graves' hyperthyroidism who received two doses of rituximab 1000 mg iv at 2 weeks at 2-week intervals. The study showed that 70% of the patients remained euthyroid after receiving rituximab treatment with significantly reduced levels of TRAb and free thyroxine over an average follow-up period of 18 months. Notable, those who responded well to treatment had low levels of TRAb before treatment [71].

M Salvi et al. conducted a double-blind RCT to compare rituximab with iv methylprednisolone in patients with active GO. The study showed better therapeutic outcomes with rituximab as compared to methylprednisolone, even after a lower rituximab dose [72]. RCT conducted by Stan MN et al. concluded that rituximab offers no additional benefit over placebo in patients with active and moderate to severe GO, however there were negligible adverse effects [73]. The effectiveness of rituximab in glucocorticoid refractory Graves' disease was demonstrated by Mitchell AL et al. in their study. The study was conducted on nine patients with refractory GO and showed a significant reduction in thyrotropin receptor antibody (TBII) and clinical activity score [74].

Following rituximab treatment (500 mg), patients typically experience significant B cell depletion (>99%) lasting 5–20 months, followed by gradual recovery [75]. Even the dose reduction to as low as 100 mg did not compromise its efficacy [72]. Rituximab treatment selectively spares plasma cells and memory B cells which are resistant to its action [75], but it clears all the lymphoid cells from thyroid tissue [76]. The remaining memory B cells and plasma cells might still produce harmful TRAb antibodies, which could explain why rituximab is not fully successful in treating Graves' hyperthyroidism. Research in type 1 diabetes patients shows that rituximab does not reset the early stages of B cell development, which is why it does not lead to lasting remission [77].

Clinical trials have identified mild infusion reactions as the most common adverse events related to rituximab therapy. Post-marketing reports have identified a potential association between rituximab treatment and immune complex-mediated adverse events, including arthralgias and gastrointestinal disturbances, such as colitis. [78]. Rituximab treatment has been associated with an elevated risk of severe infections, particularly in individuals with profound immunodeficiency or underlying malignancies [79]. Progressive multifocal leukoencephalopathy (PML) is a rare but potentially life-threatening complication predominantly observed in individuals with underlying conditions receiving concurrent immunosuppressive therapies [80]. A comprehensive 9.5-year review of repeated rituximab (RTX) courses in rheumatoid arthritis patients revealed no elevated safety risks or increased adverse event rates compared to placebo plus methotrexate [81].

Second-generation CD20-depleting agents, including ocrelizumab and ofatumumab, exhibit enhanced tolerability and reduced immunogenicity, potentially benefiting patients with Graves' disease [82, 83].

6.2 Targeting B-cell proliferation and activation through BAFF

B cell-activating factor (BAFF), a member of the tumor necrosis factor family, is indispensable for B cell development, survival, and homeostasis and modulates T cell-independent immune responses [84]. Studies have identified a significant association between the genetic variant rs2893321 and increased susceptibility to Graves' disease (GD) and autoimmune thyroid diseases (AITDs) [85], with a notable correlation with thyroid autoantibody (TAb) levels [86]. Belimumab, a human monoclonal antibody, neutralizes soluble BAFF, blocking receptor interaction and reducing autoantibody production [85]. Immunohistochemical analysis reveals increased expression of BAFF and BAFF-R in thyrocytes and infiltrating immune cells of patients with autoimmune thyroid diseases (AITD) [87]. There is an RCT undergoing to assess the efficacy of Belimumab for Graves' disease with active orbitopathy.

Clinical trials and post-marketing data confirm belimumab's safety and efficacy in SLE patients without increased risk of serious infections [88, 89]. Belimumab failed to show significant therapeutic benefit in ANCA-associated vasculitis patients [90]. Belimumab, whether used alone or with RTX, has shown effectiveness in treating SLE, significantly reducing long-term organ damage [88, 89]. Nevertheless, the UK Medicines and Healthcare Products Regulatory Agency has reported an increased risk of psychiatric events in SLE patients taking belimumab [91].

6.3 Disruption of B-cell activation or activity

6.3.1 Blocking CD40 interactions

One key cell-to-cell interaction involved in regulating adaptive immune responses is the CD40–CD154 (CD40 ligand) pathway. CD40 is found on B-cells, macrophages, and dendritic cells (DCs), while CD154 is present on activated T cells. The fact that CD40 is expressed not only on B-cells but also on antigen-presenting cells (APCs) and other cell types highlights the significance of the CD40–CD154 interaction in T-cell-mediated immune responses. This interaction plays a critical role in the development of effector functions across various CD40-expressing cells. Targeting this pathway using anti-CD154 monoclonal antibodies (mAbs) could serve as an effective therapeutic strategy for reducing inflammation, controlling autoimmune diseases, and preventing graft rejection [92].CD40, a receptor from the tumor necrosis factor family, is a key immune-modulating gene associated with susceptibility to Graves' disease (GD). In thyrocytes, CD40 primarily functions through NF-κB, with both the NF-κB1 and NF-κB2 pathways playing a role in initiating and progressing GD [93]. The CD40-CD154 interaction between B and T lymphocytes is believed to play a crucial role in the development of Graves' hyperthyroidism. It is necessary for the formation of intrathyroidal germinal centres and the maturation of the B-cell repertoire, which enables the production of harmful thyroid-stimulating antibodies.

The CD40 Kozak SNP allele, associated with Graves' disease, enhances the translation efficiency of CD40 mRNA, potentially increasing disease susceptibility [93]. Iscalimab, a fully human anti-CD40 monoclonal antibody engineered with an N297A mutation to abrogate Fcγ-dependent effector functions, demonstrated potent suppression of CD154-induced leukocyte activation in vitro [94]. Thus, iscalimab inhibits CD40 interactions without actually depleting CD40-expressing cells. The role of iscalimab has been best studied in an RCT, where it proved to be effective.

A multicenter, open-label phase II study enrolled 15 patients with Graves' disease, administering iscalimab at 10 mg/kg intravenously five times over 12 weeks. A clinical response and biochemical euthyroidism were achieved in 7/15 (47%) patients, with normalization of free and total triiodothyronine and thyroxine levels, without requirement for antithyroid drug (ATD) rescue therapy. Four of the seven responders relapsed after completing the treatment. Serum concentrations of thyrotropin receptor autoantibodies [TSH-R-Ab] significantly declined in all patients [mean 15.3 IU/L vs. 4.0 IU/L, a 66% reduction; $P < 0.001$], and TSH-R-Ab levels normalized in 4 patients [27%]. Iscalimab therapy was associated with rapid and significant reductions in serum CXCL13 concentrations ($P < 0.001$). Twelve patients (80.0%) experienced at least one adverse event, with all treatment-related AEs classified as mild or moderate and resolving by study completion [95].

6.3.2 Blocking immunoglobulin recycling [FcRn therapeutics]

Immunoglobulin G [IgG] antibodies are vital components of the adaptive immune response, designed to protect the body from infections. Compared to other immunoglobulins, immunoglobulin G (IgG) exhibits distinct characteristics, including elevated serum concentrations, prolonged half-life and transplacental transfer. These properties are expedited by interactions with the neonatal Fc receptor. FcRn's pH-dependent binding prevents IgG degradation by lysosomes. Additionally, FcRn enables the transport of IgGs across polarized cells that separate different tissue compartments, such as the endothelium and epithelium [96]. The neonatal Fc receptor (FcRn) mediates prolonged circulation of TRab IgG antibodies by recycling endocytosed molecules through lysosomal acidification and exocytosis [97]. A study conducted by N. Li et al. examined the effect of IVIG on autoantibody-mediated cutaneous bullous disease. The study concluded that administering high doses of IVIG accelerated the degradation of pathogenic IgG by saturating the MHC-like Fc receptor, neonatal Fc receptor [FcRn]. Additionally, the study found that FcRn-deficient mice were resistant to autoimmune diseases. Therefore, FcRn represents a promising therapeutic target for treating IgG-mediated autoimmune diseases [98]. Graves' disease is an IgG-mediated autoimmune disorder where accelerated antibody catabolism and a subsequent reduction in circulating pathogenic TRAb levels would be beneficial. The two most prominent drugs in this category are the Fc fragment efgartigimod and the monoclonal antibody rozanolixizumab. The development of these molecules ranges from preclinical stages to ongoing phase 3 trials, with promising results demonstrated in conditions like ITP and myasthenia gravis. IVIG exerts its immunomodulatory effects in autoimmune diseases through Fc receptor saturation and blockade. Improved binding affinity translates to reduced dosage requirements [less than 50 mg/kg compared to 1–2 g/kg body weight] [99]. Efgartigimod represents a truncated IgG1 Fc region, while rozanolixizumab is a fully humanized IgG4 monoclonal antibody directed against FcRn. The blockade of FcRn-IgG interactions by efgartigimod and rozanolixizumab inhibits IgG recycling and accelerates the removal of pathogenic IgG antibodies from circulation [100]. Efgartigimod has been investigated in patients with myasthenia gravis in a randomized phase 2 study; it showed a rapid decrease of up to 70% in total immunoglobulin G and anti-AChR autoantibody levels in 75% of subjects, compared to 25% of the placebo group proving that it may offer a future innovative approach to treat autoimmune diseases [101]. Efgartigimod was used in phase 2 study in adults with ITP, in which 38 patients were randomized. Efgartigimod's IgG-reducing effects translated to clinically meaningful improvements in platelet counts and bleeding reduction. All the studies on efgartigimod and rozanolixizumab have shown no serious adverse effects, with headache being the most frequent side effect and no treatment-related serious side effects [100, 101]. Fc and FcγR-targeting therapeutics encompass molecules that specifically interact with the Fc domain of IgG, including recombinant soluble FcγIIb receptors (e.g., valziflocept, SM101/SHP652) and monoclonal antibodies directed against Fcγ receptors [102].

6.4 TSH-specific treatment options

Graves' disease arises from the stimulation of the TSH receptor [TSHR]. Therefore, directly preventing TSHR activation and its downstream signaling would be a more effective approach in managing the disease without adversely affecting the individual's immune system. Researchers are designing therapeutic strategies to antagonize TSHR signal transduction through small molecules or neutralizing antibodies. Additionally, studies are examining the immunomodulatory effects of TSHR peptide for long-term therapeutic application. Compared to other innovative approaches in treating Graves' disease, these targeted molecules are specific and less likely to negatively impact the patient's immune system.

6.4.1 Small molecule TSHR antagonist

Small molecules acting as agonist or antagonist at TSHR can directly stimulate or inhibit TSHR signaling. Because TSHR plays an important role in the pathogenesis of thyroid disease, this could be a future potent therapy in hyperthyroidism. Susanne et al. in their study described the first small molecule ANTAG 3 by chemical modification of a previously reported TSHR antagonist, that acts as an inverse agonist properties at TSHR. It suppresses both basal and stimulated cAMP signaling; the antagonism at TSH-mediated signaling is competitive. It lowers serum-free T4 levels and thyroid gene expression [103].

VA-K-14 and S37a are the two new TSH-receptor antagonist compounds discovered. They have been found to block TSH and TRAb-induced signaling in vitro [104, 105]. Due to the structural homology between TSHR, follicle-stimulating hormone receptor, and luteinizing hormone/chorionic gonadotropin receptor, there are side effects related to the stimulation of these receptors. VA-K-14 has minor side effects related to FSH antagonism while S37a is more specific.

The compound exhibits allosteric binding to the TSH receptor, interacting at sites distinct from orthosteric binding sites of thyroid-stimulating hormone and thyroid receptor antibodies, ensuring effectiveness irrespective of TRAb concentration. They are effective orally and are suitable for long-term administration. Although human trials have not yet been conducted, these compounds hold promise as effective drugs for treating Graves' hyperthyroidism in the future [103–105].

6.4.2 TSH-blocking antibodies

Occasionally, patients with Graves' ophthalmopathy [GO] may exhibit active inflammatory eye disease despite having hypothyroidism and high titres of TRAb antibodies, which include a mix of TSHR-blocking antibodies. Some patients present with both stimulating and blocking TSHR autoantibodies in their serum, although these activities have not been separated and analyzed extensively. Nils G et al. successfully isolated and characterized two distinct TSH receptor monoclonal antibodies (Ki-70) from a single blood sample, blocking type and stimulating type [106]. Jadwiga et al. in their study discovered that M22 stimulates thyroid hormone secretion, and K1-70 inhibits thyroid hormone secretion and counters the effects of M22. K1-70 shows a promising future in treating Graves' hyperthyroidism and Graves' orbitopathy [107].

6.4.3 TSH-specific immunotherapy

Antigen-specific immunotherapy induces immune tolerance by gradual allergen exposure and increases the threshold for allergic response [108]. This therapeutic

Candidate drugs	Therapeutic mechanism	Regimen	Clinical trials
Rituximab (anti-CD 20)	Deplete B-cells by binding to CD 20 receptors on B cells.	Not available at present	Phase 2 clinical trials [70, 71]
Belimumab (anti-BAFF)	B cell activating factor (BAFF) neutralizing antibody.	Not available at present	Phase 2 trial (EudraCT 2015–002127-26)
Iscalimab (anti-CD-40 mAb)	Blocking CD 40 and CD 154 co-stimulatory pathway, attenuating B cell activation.	10 mg/kg IV over 12 weeks	Phase II trial [95]
Efgartigimod Rozanolixizumab	Block FcRn-IgG interactions, inhibiting IgG recycling and accelerating removal of pathogenic IgG.	50 mg/kg	Preclinical stages to Phase 3 trials [99–101]
VA-K-14 and S37a (TSH receptor antagonist molecule)	Competitive antagonism of TSH mediated signaling.	—	Preclinical [103–105]
K1–70 (Anti-TRAb mAb)	Human monoclonal antibody blocking TSH- receptor.	Single IM or IV injection at different doses (0.2–150 mg) have been tested	Phase 1 clinical trial [NCT02904330]
ATX-GD-59	Induces immune tolerance by exposure to low dose antigen.	Ten doses intradermally over 18 weeks' time.	Phase 1 clinical trial [110]

Table 1.
Graves' disease—Novel treatments and their various developmental stages.

strategy aims to restore immune homeostasis by inducing tolerance to self-antigen. This is done by administering synthetic peptides called "apitopes" [antigen-processing independent epitopes] that mimic naturally processed CD4+ T cell epitopes. However, concerns exist regarding the potential for administering antigens to a susceptible individual may exacerbate disease severity. Peptide-based epitopes showed a promising future for targeted therapy in type 1 diabetes (proinsulin peptides) and multiple sclerosis (myelin basic protein peptides) [108, 109]. New hope for Graves' disease patients is ATX-GD-59. It is a combination of two immunodominant receptors from humans. In phase 1 study, it showed a 70% response rate in adult with untreated Graves' disease. There was normalization of fT3 levels in 5 patients. It was well tolerated with minor injection site reactions [110].

Targeted immunotherapy is the future hope for patients with Graves' disease. It is an approach that reduces the risk of generalized immunosuppression. There is a potential for long-term remission. The ongoing research on immunotherapy aims to optimize safety and efficacy (**Table 1**).

Figure 2 summarizes a therapeutic strategy for Graves' hyperthyroidism and **Figure 3** gives schematic repression of the mechanism of action of emerging therapies (**Figure 3**).

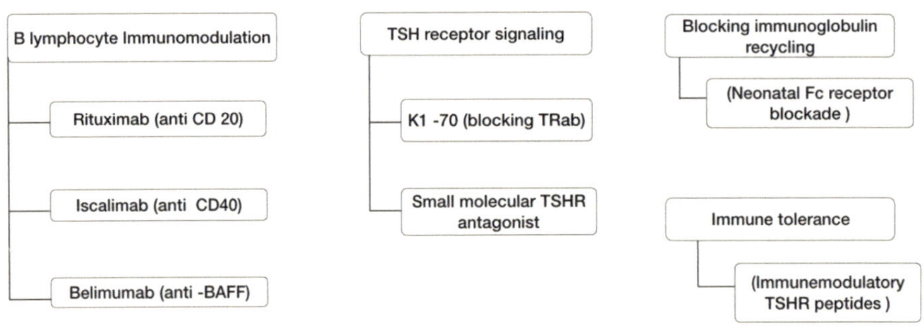

Figure 2.
Illustration of emerging therapies for the treatment of Graves' disease.

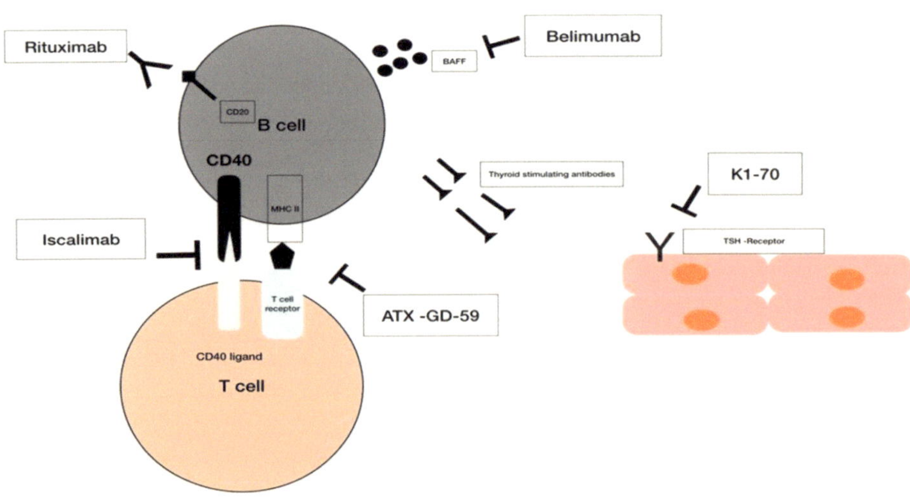

Figure 3.
Schematic representation of emerging therapeutic strategies for Graves' hyperthyroidism management.

7. Limitations

Though the above approaches seem attractive, they are not without limitations. The main limitation is cost, also since these drugs suppress immunity, they cannot be used in immunocompromised patients. Their efficacy in reducing the risk of hypothyroidism, goiter size and relapse of goiter is unclear.

8. Conclusions

The available diagnostic modalities and treatment options, which include surgery, radioiodine and antithyroid drugs, remained unchanged since late 1940. New treatments for thyroid issues are being developed, using various methods such as biologics, small molecules, and peptides to modulate the immune system. These therapies are in different stages of research, and some will soon be available in clinics. These new treatments might make current methods like radioiodine therapy and thyroid surgery less common and eventually obsolete. However, it's important to weigh the benefits of maintaining normal thyroid function without ongoing medication against the risks, such as weakening the immune system. Future research should aim to find the best ways to combine traditional and new therapies for the most effective treatment.

Author details

Ruchi Agrawal and Shahnaz Ahmad*
Department of Endocrinology, Government Medical College Srinagar Jammu and Kashmir, India

*Address all correspondence to: mirdrshani@gmail.com

References

[1] Tomer Y. Mechanisms of autoimmune thyroid diseases: From genetics to epigenetics. Annual Review of Pathology. 2014;**9**:147-156. DOI: 10.1146/annurev-pathol-012513-104713

[2] Brix TH, Kyvik KO, Christensen K, Hegedüs L. Evidence for a major role of heredity in Graves' disease: A population-based study of two Danish twin cohorts. The Journal of Clinical Endocrinology and Metabolism. 2001;**86**(2):930-934. DOI: 10.1210/jcem.86.2.7242

[3] Zimmermann MB, Boelaert K. Iodine deficiency and thyroid disorders. The Lancet Diabetes and Endocrinology. 2015;**3**(4):286-295. DOI: 10.1016/S2213-8587(14)70225-6. Epub 2015 Jan 13

[4] Tellez M, Cooper J, Edmonds C. Graves' ophthalmopathy in relation to cigarette smoking and ethnic origin. Clinical Endocrinology. 1992;**36**(3):291-294. DOI: 10.1111/j.1365-2265.1992.tb01445.x

[5] Bahn RS. Graves' ophthalmopathy. The New England Journal of Medicine. 2010;**362**(8):726-738. DOI: 10.1056/NEJMra0905750

[6] Limbach M, Saare M, Tserel L, Kisand K, Eglit T, Sauer S, et al. Epigenetic profiling in CD4+ and CD8+ T cells from Graves' disease patients reveals changes in genes associated with T cell receptor signaling. Journal of Autoimmunity. 2016;**67**:46-56. DOI: 10.1016/j.jaut.2015.09.006

[7] Coles AJ, Wing M, Smith S, Coraddu F, Greer S, Taylor C, et al. Pulsed monoclonal antibody treatment and autoimmune thyroid disease in multiple sclerosis. Lancet. 1999;**354**(9191):1691-1695. DOI: 10.1016/S0140-6736(99)02429-0

[8] Effraimidis G, Wiersinga WM. Mechanisms in endocrinology: Autoimmune thyroid disease: Old and new players. European Journal of Endocrinology. 2014;**170**(6):R241-R252. DOI: 10.1530/EJE-14-0047. Epub 2014 Mar 7

[9] Rapoport B, McLachlan SM. Graves' hyperthyroidism is antibody mediated but is predominantly a Th1-type cytokine disease. The Journal of Clinical Endocrinology and Metabolism. 2014;**99**(11):4060-4061

[10] Weetman AP, Yateman ME, Ealey PA, Black CM, Reimer CB, Williams RC Jr, et al. Thyroid-stimulating antibody activity between different immunoglobulin G subclasses. The Journal of Clinical Investigation. 1990;**86**(3):723-727. DOI: 10.1172/JCI114768

[11] Zakarija M. Immunochemical characterization of the thyroid stimulating antibody (TSAb) of Graves' disease: Evidence for restricted heterogeneity. Journal of Clinical & Laboratory Immunology. 1983;**10**(2):77-85

[12] Morshed SA, Latif R, Davies TF. Characterization of thyrotropin receptor antibody-induced signaling cascades. Endocrinology. 2009;**150**(1):519-529. DOI: 10.1210/en.2008-0878. Epub 2008 Aug 21

[13] Rapoport B, Aliesky HA, Chen CR, McLachlan SM. Evidence that TSH receptor A-subunit multimers, not monomers, drive antibody affinity maturation in Graves' disease. The Journal of Clinical Endocrinology and Metabolism. 2015;**100**(6):E871-E875. DOI: 10.1210/jc.2015-1528. Epub 2015 Apr 9

[14] Pritchard J, Han R, Horst N, Cruikshank WW, Smith TJ. Immunoglobulin activation of T cell chemoattractant expression in fibroblasts from patients with Graves' disease is mediated through the insulin-like growth factor I receptor pathway. Journal of Immunology. 2003;**170**(12):6348-6354. DOI: 10.4049/jimmunol.170.12.6348

[15] McLachlan SM, Rapoport B. Breaking tolerance to thyroid antigens: Changing concepts in thyroid autoimmunity. Endocrine Reviews. 2014;**35**(1):59-105

[16] Klatka M et al. Th17 and Treg cells in adolescents with graves' dis- ease. Impact of treatment with methimazole on these cell subsets. Autoimmunity. 2014;**47**(3):201-211

[17] Murakami M et al. Thymic hyperplasia in patients with Graves' disease. Identification of thyrotropin receptors in human thymus. The Journal of Clinical Investigation. 1996;**98**(10):2228-2234

[18] Stefan M et al. Genetic-epigenetic dysregulation of thymic TSH receptor gene expression triggers thyroid autoimmunity. Proceedings of the National Academy of Sciences of the United States of America. 2014;**111**(34):12562-12567

[19] Vignali DA, Collison LW, Workman CJ. How regulatory T cells work. Nature Reviews. Immunology. 2008;**8**(7):523-532. DOI: 10.1038/nri2343

[20] Bossowski A et al. Decreased proportions of CD4 + IL17+/CD4 + CD25 + CD127- and CD4 + IL17+/CD4 + CD25 + CD127 - FoxP3+ T cells in children with autoimmune thyroid diseases (.). Autoimmunity. 2016;**49**(5):320-328

[21] Fang S et al. Regulation of orbital fibrosis and adipogenesis by pathogenic Th17 cells in Graves' orbitopathy. The Journal of Clinical Endocrinology and Metabolism. 2017;**102**(11):4273-4283

[22] Wang Z et al. Integrative analysis of mRNA and miRNA array data reveals the suppression of retinoic acid pathway in regulatory T cells of Graves' disease. The Journal of Clinical Endocrinology and Metabolism. 2014;**99**(12):E2620-E2627

[23] Yuan Q et al. Low regulatory T cell and high IL-17 mRNA expression in a mouse Graves' disease model. Journal of Endocrinological Investigation. 2017;**40**(4):397-407

[24] Nagata K, Nakayama Y, Higaki K, Ochi M, Kanai K, Matsushita M, et al. Reactivation of persistent Epstein-Barr virus (EBV) causes secretion of thyrotropin receptor antibodies (TRAbs) in EBV-infected B lymphocytes with TRAbs on their surface. Autoimmunity. 2015;**48**(5):328-335. DOI: 10.3109/08916934.2015.1022163. Epub 2015 Mar 11

[25] Armengol MP, Cardoso-Schmidt CB, Fernández M, Ferrer X, Pujol-Borrell R, Juan M. Chemokines determine local lymphoneogenesis and a reduction of circulating CXCR4+ T and CCR7 B and T lymphocytes in thyroid autoimmune diseases. Journal of Immunology. 2003;**170**(12):6320-6328. DOI: 10.4049/jimmunol.170.12.6320

[26] Hanafusa T, Pujol-Borrell R, Chiovato L, Russell RC, Doniach D, Bottazzo GF. Aberrant expression of HLA-DR antigen on thyrocytes in Graves' disease: Relevance for autoimmunity. Lancet. 1983;**2**(8359):1111-1115. DOI: 10.1016/s0140-6736(83)90628-1

[27] Faure GC, Bensoussan-Lejzerowicz D, Bene MC, Aubert V, Leclere J. Coexpression of CD40 and class II antigen HLA-DR in Graves'

disease thyroid epithelial cells. Clinical Immunology and Immunopathology. 1997;**84**(2):212-215. DOI: 10.1006/clin.1997.4391

[28] Smith TJ, Sciaky D, Phipps RP, Jennings TA. CD40 expression in human thyroid tissue: Evidence for involvement of multiple cell types in autoimmune and neoplastic diseases. Thyroid. 1999;**9**(8):749-755. DOI: 10.1089/thy.1999.9.749

[29] Rapoport B, McLachlan SM. The thyrotropin receptor in Graves' disease. Thyroid. 2007;**17**(10):911-922. DOI: 10.1089/thy.2007.0170

[30] Laurberg P, Wallin G, Tallstedt L, Abraham-Nordling M, Lundell G, Tørring O. TSH-receptor autoimmunity in Graves' disease after therapy with anti-thyroid drugs, surgery, or radioiodine: A 5-year prospective randomized study. European Journal of Endocrinology. 2008;**158**(1):69-75. DOI: 10.1530/EJE-07-0450

[31] Morshed SA, Davies TF. Graves' disease mechanisms: The role of stimulating, blocking, and cleavage region TSH receptor antibod- ies. Hormone and Metabolic Research. 2015;**47**(10):727-734

[32] Morshed SA, Latif R, Davies TF. Characterization of thyrotro-pin receptor antibody-induced signaling cascades. Endocrinology. 2009;**150**(1):519-529

[33] LiVolsi VA, Baloch ZW. The pathology of hyperthyroidism. Front Endocrinology (Lausanne). 2018;**9**:737. DOI: 10.3389/fendo.2018.00737

[34] Dimai HP, Ramschak-Schwarzer S, Lax S, et al. Hyperthyroidism of Graves' disease: Evidence for only unilateral involvement of the thyroid gland in a 31-year-old female patient. Journal of Endocrinological Investigation. 1999;**22**:215-219. DOI: 10.1007/BF03343545

[35] Franklyn JA, Boelaert K. Thyrotoxicosis. Lancet. 2012;**379**(9821):1155-1166. DOI: 10.1016/S0140-6736(11)60782-4. Epub 2012 Mar 5

[36] Bartalena L, Tanda ML. Clinical practice. Graves' ophthalmopathy. The New England Journal of Medicine. 2009;**360**(10):994-1001. DOI: 10.1056/NEJMcp0806317

[37] Fatourechi V. Thyroid dermopathy and acropachy. Best Practice & Research. Clinical Endocrinology & Metabolism. 2012;**26**(4):553-565. DOI: 10.1016/j.beem.2011.10.001. Epub 2012 May 22

[38] Boelaert K, Torlinska B, Holder RL, Franklyn JA. Older subjects with hyperthyroidism present with a paucity of symptoms and signs: A large cross-sectional study. The Journal of Clinical Endocrinology and Metabolism. 2010;**95**(6):2715-2726. DOI: 10.1210/jc.2009-2495. Epub 2010 Apr 14

[39] Bartalena L, Pinchera A, Marcocci C. Management of Graves' ophthalmopathy: Reality and perspectives. Endocrine Reviews. 2000;**21**(2):168-199. DOI: 10.1210/edrv.21.2.0393

[40] Parameswaran R, de Jong MC, Kit JLW, Sek K, Nam TQ, Thang TV, et al. 2021 Asia-Pacific graves' disease consortium survey of clinical practice patterns in the management of Graves' disease. Endocrine. 2023;**79**(1):135-142. DOI: 10.1007/s12020-022-03193-7. Epub 2022 Sep 21

[41] Burch HB, Burman KD, Cooper DS. A 2011 survey of clinical practice patterns in the management of Graves'

disease. The Journal of Clinical Endocrinology and Metabolism. 2012;**97**(12):4549-4558. DOI: 10.1210/jc.2012-2802. Epub 2012 Oct 5

[42] Bahn RS et al. Hyperthyroidism and other causes of thyrotoxicosis: Management guidelines of the American Thyroid Association and American Association of Clinical Endocrinologists. Thyroid. 2011;**21**:593-646

[43] Ross DS, Burch HB, Cooper DS, Greenlee MC, Laurberg P, Maia AL, et al. 2016 American Thyroid Association guidelines for diagnosis and management of hyperthyroidism and other causes of thyrotoxicosis. Thyroid. 2016;**26**(10):1343-1421. DOI: 10.1089/thy.2016.0229. Erratum in: Thyroid. 2017 Nov;27(11):1462. doi: 10.1089/thy.2016.0229.correx

[44] Smith BR, Hall R. Thyroid-stimulating immunoglobulins in Graves' disease. Lancet. 1974;**304**(7878):427-430. DOI: 10.1016/S0140-6736(74)91791-7

[45] Zöphel K, Roggenbuck D, Schott M. Clinical review about TRAb assay's history. Autoimmunity Reviews. 2010;**9**(10):695-700. DOI: 10.1016/j.autrev.2010.05.021. Epub 2010 Jun 4

[46] Sanders J, Evans M, Betterle C, Sanders P, Bhardwaja A, Young S, et al. A human monoclonal autoantibody to the thyrotropin receptor with thyroid-stimulating blocking activity. Thyroid. 2008;**18**(7):735-746. DOI: 10.1089/thy.2007.0327

[47] Schott M, Hermsen D, Broecker-Preuss M, Casati M, Mas JC, Eckstein A, et al. Clinical value of the first automated TSH receptor autoantibody assay for the diagnosis of Graves' disease (GD): An international multicentre trial. Clinical Endocrinology. 2009;**71**(4):566-573. DOI: 10.1111/j.1365-2265.2008.03512.x. Epub 2008 Dec 17

[48] Tozzoli R, Bagnasco M, Giavarina D, Bizzaro N. TSH receptor autoantibody immunoassay in patients with Graves' disease: Improvement of diagnostic accuracy over different generations of methods. Systematic Review and Meta-Analysis. Autoimmun Review. 2012;**12**(2):107-113. DOI: 10.1016/j.autrev.2012.07.003. Epub 2012 Jul 7

[49] Bogazzi F, Vitti P. Could improved ultrasound and power Doppler replace thyroidal radioiodine uptake to assess thyroid disease? Nature Clinical Practice. Endocrinology & Metabolism. 2008;**4**(2):70-71. DOI: 10.1038/ncpendmet0692. Epub 2007 Nov 6

[50] Vitti P, Rago T, Mazzeo S, Brogioni S, Lampis M, De Liperi A, et al. Thyroid blood flow evaluation by color-flow Doppler sonography distinguishes Graves' disease from Hashimoto's thyroiditis. Journal of Endocrinological Investigation. 1995;**18**(11):857-861. DOI: 10.1007/BF03349833

[51] Cappelli C, Pirola I, De Martino E, Agosti B, Delbarba A, Castellano M, et al. The role of imaging in Graves' disease: A cost-effectiveness analysis. European Journal of Radiology. 2008;**65**(1):99-103. DOI: 10.1016/j.ejrad.2007.03.015. Epub 2007 Apr 24

[52] Boi F, Loy M, Piga M, Serra A, Atzeni F, Mariotti S. The usefulness of conventional and echo colour Doppler sonography in the differential diagnosis of toxic multinodular goitres. European Journal of Endocrinology. 2000;**143**(3):339-346. DOI: 10.1530/eje.0.1430339

[53] Kurita S, Sakurai M, Kita Y, Ota T, Ando H, Kaneko S, et al. Measurement of thyroid blood flow area is useful for diagnosing the cause of thyrotoxicosis. Thyroid. 2005;**15**(11):1249-1252. DOI: 10.1089/thy.2005.15.1249

[54] Bartalena L. Diagnosis and management of Graves' disease: A global overview. Nature Reviews. Endocrinology. 2013;**9**(12):724-734. DOI: 10.1038/nrendo.2013.193. Epub 2013 Oct 15

[55] Davidson B, Soodak M, Neary JT, Strout HV, Kieffer JD, Mover H, et al. The irreversible inactivation of thyroid peroxidase by methylmercaptoimidazole, thiouracil, and propylthiouracil In vitro and its relationship to In vivo findings. Endocrinology. 1978;**103**(3):871-882. DOI: 10.1210/endo-103-3-871

[56] Cooper DS. Antithyroid drugs in the management of patients with Graves' disease: An evidence-based approach to therapeutic controversies. The Journal of Clinical Endocrinology and Metabolism. 2003;**88**(8):3474-3481. DOI: 10.1210/jc.2003-030185

[57] Jansson R, Dahlberg PA, Lindström B. International journal of clinical pharmacology. Therapy, and Toxicology. 1983;**21**(10):505-510

[58] Kahaly GJ. Management of Graves' thyroidal and Extrathyroidal disease: An update. The Journal of Clinical Endocrinology and Metabolism. 2020;**105**(12):3704-3720. DOI: 10.1210/clinem/dgaa646

[59] Starling S. Long-term treatment outcomes for Graves' disease. Nature Reviews. Endocrinology. 2019;**15**(11):628. DOI: 10.1038/s41574-019-0268-5

[60] Masiello E, Veronesi G, Gallo D, Premoli P, Bianconi E, Rosetti S, et al. Antithyroid drug treatment for Graves' disease: Baseline predictive models of relapse after treatment for a patient-tailored management. Journal of Endocrinological Investigation. 2018;**41**(12):1425-1432. DOI: 10.1007/s40618-018-0918-9. Epub 2018 Jun 26

[61] El Kawkgi OM, Ross DS, Stan MN. Comparison of long-term Antithyroid drugs versus radioactive iodine or surgery for Graves' disease: A review of the literature. Clinical Endocrinology. 2021;**95**(1):3-12. DOI: 10.1111/cen.14374

[62] Jørgensen CU. JBMR Plus. 2021;**5**(4). Published online 2021 Mar 16. DOI: 10.1002/jbm4.10479

[63] Tabriz N, Muehlbeyer S, Weyhe D, Uslar V. Risk factors for recurrent laryngeal nerve palsy in thyroid surgery: A single center experience of 1147 procedures with intermittent intraoperative Neuromonitoring. Journal of Personalized Medicine. 2024;**14**:714. DOI: 10.3390/jpm14070714

[64] Rastogi I, Jeon D, Moseman JE, Muralidhar A, Potluri HK, McNeel DG. Role of B cells as antigen presenting cells. Frontiers in Immunology. 2022;**13**:954936. DOI: 10.3389/fimmu.2022.954936

[65] Pichurin P, Aliesky H, Chen CR, Nagayama Y, Rapoport B, McLachlan SM. Thyrotrophin receptor-specific memory T cell responses require normal B cells in a murine model of Graves' disease. Clinical and Experimental Immunology. 2003;**134**(3):396-402. DOI: 10.1111/j.1365-2249.2003.02322.x

[66] Gürcan HM, Keskin DB, Stern JN, Nitzberg MA, Shekhani H, Ahmed AR. A review of the current use of rituximab in autoimmune diseases. International Immunopharmacology. 2009;**9**(1):10-25. DOI: 10.1016/j.intimp.2008.10.004. Epub 2008 Nov 8

[67] Cerny T, Borisch B, Introna M, Johnson P, Rose AL. Mechanism of action of rituximab. Anti-Cancer Drugs. 2002;**13**(Suppl 2):S3-S10. DOI: 10.1097/00001813-200211002-00002

[68] Cho A, Bradley B, Kauffman R, Priyamvada L, Kovalenkov Y, Feldman R, et al. Robust memory responses against influenza vaccination in pemphigus patients previously treated with rituximab. JCI Insight. 2017;**2**(12):e93222. DOI: 10.1172/jci.insight.93222

[69] Cheetham TD, Cole M, Abinun M, Allahabadia A, Barratt T, Davies JH, et al. Adjuvant rituximab-exploratory trial in Young people with Graves' disease. The Journal of Clinical Endocrinology and Metabolism. 2022;**107**(3):743-754. DOI: 10.1210/clinem/dgab763

[70] El Fassi D, Banga JP, Gilbert JA, Padoa C, Hegedüs L, Nielsen CH. Treatment of Graves' disease with rituximab specifically reduces the production of thyroid stimulating autoantibodies. Clinical Immunology. 2009;**130**(3):252-258. DOI: 10.1016/j.clim.2008.09.007. Epub 2008 Oct 28

[71] Heemstra KA, Toes RE, Sepers J, Pereira AM, Corssmit EP, Huizinga TW, et al. Rituximab in relapsing Graves' disease, a phase II study. European Journal of Endocrinology. 2008;**159**(5):609-615. DOI: 10.1530/EJE-08-0084. Epub 2008 Jul 15

[72] Salvi M, Vannucchi G, Currò N, Campi I, Covelli D, Dazzi D, et al. Efficacy of B-cell targeted therapy with rituximab in patients with active moderate to severe Graves' orbitopathy: A randomized controlled study. The Journal of Clinical Endocrinology and Metabolism. 2015;**100**(2):422-431. DOI: 10.1210/jc.2014-3014. Epub 2014 Dec 15

[73] Stan MN, Salvi M. Management of endocrine disease: Rituximab therapy for Graves' orbitopathy—Lessons from randomized control trials. European Journal of Endocrinology. 2017;**176**(2):R101-R109. DOI: 10.1530/EJE-16-0552. Epub 2016 Oct 19

[74] Mitchell C, Crayne CB, Cron RQ. Patterns of B cell repletion following rituximab therapy in a pediatric rheumatology cohort. ACR Open Rheumatology. 2019;**1**(8):527-532. DOI: 10.1002/acr2.11074

[75] Leandro MJ, Cambridge G, Ehrenstein MR, Edwards JC. Reconstitution of peripheral blood B cells after depletion with rituximab in patients with rheumatoid arthritis. Arthritis and Rheumatism. 2006;**54**(2):613-620. DOI: 10.1002/art.21617

[76] El Fassi D, Nielsen CH, Bonnema SJ, Hasselbalch HC, Hegedüs L. B lymphocyte depletion with the monoclonal antibody rituximab in Graves' disease: A controlled pilot study. The Journal of Clinical Endocrinology and Metabolism. 2007;**92**(5):1769-1772. DOI: 10.1210/jc.2006-2388. Epub 2007 Feb 6

[77] Chamberlain N, Massad C, Oe T, Cantaert T, Herold KC, Meffre E. Rituximab does not reset defective early B cell tolerance checkpoints. The Journal of Clinical Investigation. 2016;**126**(1):282-287. DOI: 10.1172/JCI83840. Epub 2015 Dec 7

[78] El Fassi D, Nielsen CH, Junker P, Hasselbalch HC, Hegedüs L. Systemic adverse events following rituximab therapy in patients with Graves' disease. Journal of Endocrinological Investigation. 2011;**34**(7):e163-e167. DOI: 10.3275/7411. Epub 2010 Dec 15

[79] Gea-Banacloche JC. Rituximab-associated infections. Seminars in Hematology. 2010;**47**(2):187-198. DOI: 10.1053/j.seminhematol.2010.01.002

[80] Berger JR, Malik V, Lacey S, Brunetta P, Lehane PB. Progressive

multifocal leukoencephalopathy in rituximab-treated rheumatic diseases: A rare event. Journal of Neurovirology. 2018;**24**(3):323-331. DOI: 10.1007/s13365-018-0615-7. Epub 2018 Mar 5. Erratum in: J Neurovirol. 2018;24(3):332. doi: 10.1007/s13365-018-0637-1

[81] van Vollenhoven RF, Emery P, Bingham CO 3rd, Keystone EC, Fleischmann RM, Furst DE, et al. Long-term safety of rituximab in rheumatoid arthritis: 9.5-year follow-up of the global clinical trial programme with a focus on adverse events of interest in RA patients. Annals of the Rheumatic Diseases. 2013;**72**(9):1496-1502. DOI: 10.1136/annrheumdis-2012-201956. Epub 2012 Nov 7

[82] Du FH, Mills EA, Mao-Draayer Y. Next-generation anti-CD20 monoclonal antibodies in autoimmune disease treatment. Auto Immun Highlights. 2017;**8**(1):12. DOI: 10.1007/s13317-017-0100-y

[83] Bar-Or A, Grove RA, Austin DJ, Tolson JM, VanMeter SA, Lewis EW, et al. Subcutaneous ofatumumab in patients with relapsing-remitting multiple sclerosis: The MIRROR study. Neurology. 2018;**90**(20):e1805-e1814. DOI: 10.1212/WNL.0000000000005516. Epub 2018 Apr 25. Erratum in: Neurology. 2018;91(11):538. doi: 10.1212/WNL.0000000000005929

[84] Mackay F, Browning JL. BAFF: A fundamental survival factor for B cells. Nature Reviews. Immunology. 2002;**2**(7):465-475. DOI: 10.1038/nri844

[85] Lane LC, Allinson KR, Campbell K, Bhatnagar I, Ingoe L, Razvi S, et al. Analysis of BAFF gene polymorphisms in UK Graves' disease patients. Clinical Endocrinology. 2019;**90**(1):170-174. DOI: 10.1111/cen.13872. Epub 2018 Nov 5

[86] Lin JD, Wang YH, Fang WF, Hsiao CJ, Chagnaadorj A, Lin YF, et al. Serum BAFF and thyroid autoantibodies in autoimmune thyroid disease. Clinica Chimica Acta. 2016;**462**:96-102. DOI: 10.1016/j.cca.2016.09.004. Epub 2016 Sep 8

[87] Campi I, Tosi D, Rossi S, Vannucchi G, Covelli D, Colombo F, et al. B cell activating factor (BAFF) and BAFF receptor expression in autoimmune and nonautoimmune thyroid diseases. Thyroid. 2015;**25**(9):1043-1049. DOI: 10.1089/thy.2015.0029. Epub 2015 Aug 13

[88] Stohl W, Hiepe F, Latinis KM, Thomas M, Scheinberg MA, Clarke A, et al. Belimumab reduces autoantibodies, normalizes low complement levels, and reduces select B cell populations in patients with systemic lupus erythematosus. Arthritis and Rheumatism. 2012;**64**(7):2328-2337. DOI: 10.1002/art.34400

[89] Navarra SV, Guzmán RM, Gallacher AE, Hall S, Levy RA, Jimenez RE, et al. Efficacy and safety of belimumab in patients with active systemic lupus erythematosus: A randomised, placebo-controlled, phase 3 trial. Lancet. 2011;**377**(9767):721-731. DOI: 10.1016/S0140-6736(10)61354-2. Epub 2011 Feb 4

[90] Jayne D, Blockmans D, Luqmani R, Moiseev S, Ji B, Green Y, et al. Efficacy and safety of Belimumab and azathioprine for maintenance of remission in Antineutrophil cytoplasmic antibody-associated Vasculitis: A randomized controlled Study. Arthritis Rheumatology. 2019;**71**(6):952-963. DOI: 10.1002/art.40802. Epub 2019 Apr 16

[91] Xie W, Huang H, Zhan S, Zhang Z. Risk of psychiatric disorders and

all-cause mortality with belimumab therapy in patients with systemic lupus erythematosus: A meta-analysis of randomised controlled trials. Lupus Science and Medicine. 2021;**8**(1):e000534. DOI: 10.1136/lupus-2021-000534

[92] Toubi E. B cells: A main player in the development of autoimmunity. In: Perricone C, Shoenfeld Y, editors. Mosaic of Autoimmunity. Cambridge, Massachusetts, USA: Academic Press; 2019. pp. 15-19. ISBN: 9780128143070

[93] Lee HJ, Lombardi A, Stefan M, Li CW, Inabnet WB 3rd, Owen RP, et al. CD40 signaling in Graves' disease is mediated through canonical and noncanonical thyroidal nuclear factor κB activation. Endocrinology. 2017;**158**(2):410-418. DOI: 10.1210/en.2016-1609

[94] Ristov J, Espie P, Ulrich P, Sickert D, Flandre T, Dimitrova M, et al. Characterization of the in vitro and in vivo properties of CFZ533, a blocking and non-depleting anti-CD40 monoclonal antibody. American Journal of Transplantation. 2018;**18**(12):2895-2904. DOI: 10.1111/ajt.14872. Epub 2018 May 24

[95] Kahaly GJ, Stan MN, Frommer L, Gergely P, Colin L, Amer A, et al. A novel anti-CD40 monoclonal antibody, iscalimab, for control of Graves' hyperthyroidism-a proof-of-concept trial. The Journal of Clinical Endocrinology and Metabolism. 2020;**105**(3):dgz013. DOI: 10.1210/clinem/dgz013

[96] Pyzik M, Sand KMK, Hubbard JJ, Andersen JT, Sandlie I, Blumberg RS. The neonatal Fc receptor (FcRn): A misnomer? Frontiers in Immunology. 2019;**10**:1540. DOI: 10.3389/fimmu.2019.01540

[97] Ramdani Y, Lamamy J, Watier H, Gouilleux-Gruart V. Monoclonal antibody engineering and design to modulate FcRn activities: A comprehensive review. International Journal of Molecular Sciences. 2022;**23**(17):9604. DOI: 10.3390/ijms23179604

[98] Li N, Culton D, Diaz LA, Liu Z. Modes of action of intravenous immunoglobulin in bullous pemphigoid. The Journal of Investigative Dermatology. 2018;**138**(6):1249-1251. DOI: 10.1016/j.jid.2018.02.020

[99] Yu Z, Lennon VA. Mechanism of intravenous immune globulin therapy in antibody-mediated autoimmune diseases. The New England Journal of Medicine. 1999;**340**(3):227-228. DOI: 10.1056/NEJM199901213400311

[100] Newland AC, Sánchez-González B, Rejtő L, Egyed M, Romanyuk N, Godar M, et al. Phase 2 study of efgartigimod, a novel FcRn antagonist, in adult patients with primary immune thrombocytopenia. American Journal of Hematology. 2020 Feb;**95**(2):178-187. DOI: 10.1002/ajh.25680. Epub 2019 Dec 10

[101] Howard JF Jr, Bril V, Vu T, Karam C, Peric S, Margania T, et al. Safety, efficacy, and tolerability of efgartigimod in patients with generalised myasthenia gravis (ADAPT): A multicentre, randomised, placebo-controlled, phase 3 trial. Lancet Neurology. 2021;**20**(7):526-536. DOI: 10.1016/S1474-4422(21)00159-9. Erratum in: Lancet Neurol. 2021;20(8):e5. doi: 10.1016/S1474-4422(21)00216-7

[102] Zuercher AW, Spirig R, Baz Morelli A, Rowe T, Käsermann F. Next-generation fc receptor-targeting biologics for autoimmune diseases. Autoimmunity Reviews. 2019;**18**(10):102366.

DOI: 10.1016/j.autrev.2019.102366. Epub 2019 Aug 9

[103] Neumann S, Nir EA, Eliseeva E, Huang W, Marugan J, Xiao J, et al. A selective TSH receptor antagonist inhibits stimulation of thyroid function in female mice. Endocrinology. 2014;**155**(1):310-314. DOI: 10.1210/en.2013-1835. Epub 2013 Dec 4

[104] Latif R, Realubit RB, Karan C, Mezei M, Davies TF. TSH receptor signaling abrogation by a novel small molecule. Front Endocrinology (Lausanne). 2016;7:130. DOI: 10.3389/fendo.2016.00130

[105] Marcinkowski P, Hoyer I, Specker E, Furkert J, Rutz C, Neuenschwander M, et al. A new highly thyrotropin receptor-selective small-molecule antagonist with potential for the treatment of Graves' orbitopathy. Thyroid. 2019;**29**(1):111-123. DOI: 10.1089/thy.2018.0349. Epub 2018 Dec 15

[106] Morgenthaler NG, Ho SC, Minich WB. Stimulating and blocking thyroid-stimulating hormone (TSH) receptor autoantibodies from patients with Graves' disease and autoimmune hypothyroidism have very similar concentration, TSH receptor affinity, and binding sites. The Journal of Clinical Endocrinology & Metabolism. 2007;**92**(3):1058-1065. DOI: 10.1210/jc.2006-2213

[107] Furmaniak J, Sanders J, Young S, Kabelis K, Sanders P, Evans M, et al. In vivo effects of a human thyroid-stimulating monoclonal autoantibody (M22) and a human thyroid-blocking autoantibody (K1-70). Auto Immun Highlights. 2011;**3**(1):19-25. DOI: 10.1007/s13317-011-0025-9

[108] Alhadj Ali M, Liu YF, Arif S, Tatovic D, Shariff H, Gibson VB, et al. Metabolic and immune effects of immunotherapy with proinsulin peptide in human new-onset type 1 diabetes. Science Translational Medicine. 2017;**9**(402):eaaf7779. DOI: 10.1126/scitranslmed.aaf7779

[109] Chataway J, De Angelis F, Connick P, Parker RA, Plantone D, Doshi A, et al. Efficacy of three neuroprotective drugs in secondary progressive multiple sclerosis (MS-SMART): A phase 2b, multiarm, double-blind, randomised placebo-controlled trial. Lancet Neurology. 2020;**19**(3):214-225. DOI: 10.1016/S1474-4422(19)30485-5. Epub 2020 Jan 22

[110] Pearce SHS, Dayan C, Wraith DC, Barrell K, Olive N, Jansson L, et al. Antigen-specific immunotherapy with thyrotropin receptor peptides in Graves' hyperthyroidism: A phase I Study. Thyroid. 2019;**29**(7):1003-1011. DOI: 10.1089/thy.2019.0036. Epub 2019 Jun 13

Chapter 4

Computed Tomography (CT) Scan of the Orbit in Grave's Disease

Shervin Sharifkashani

Abstract

Graves' disease is the most common autoimmune disorder of the thyroid gland, and ophthalmopathy is one of the most common complications of the disease. The major morbidities of ophthalmopathy are sight-threatening dysthyroid optic neuropathy (DON), proptosis, strabismus, and diplopia. The main imaging modalities for the evaluation of Grave's ophthalmopathy are the orbit computed tomography scan (CT scan) and orbit magnetic resonance imaging (MRI), which, along with clinical and laboratory findings, help predict, monitor, and follow up after proper medical or surgical management. The benefits of the orbit CT scan are cost-effectiveness, ready-to-access, fast imaging, and simultaneous imaging evaluation of both soft tissue and bony orbits. The orbital apex crowding is the main indication of orbit CT scan and, consequently, decompression surgery in moderate-to-severe inactive ophthalmopathy in our tertiary referral hospital. The MRI can demonstrate the extraocular muscle edema on T2-weighted, short tau inversion recovery (STIR), and/or turbo inversion recovery magnitude (TIRM) images in active cases, which is useful for medical treatment. The objective of this chapter is to introduce the technique, indications, and clinically useful orbit CT scan findings in Graves' ophthalmopathy before and after decompression surgery, which will be discussed in detail based on our experience and relevant medical literature.

Keywords: CT scan, extraocular muscles, proptosis, lacrimal gland, orbital fat, bone remodeling, prolapse, exophthalmos, computed tomography, Grave's disease, ophthalmopathy, orbitopathy, decompression surgery

1. Introduction

Graves' disease is a thyroid gland autoimmune disorder due to anti-thyroid-stimulating hormone receptor (TSH-R) antibodies. The risk of the disease is higher in women than men (3 versus 0.5%) between 30 and 60 years of age and is the most common cause of hyperthyroidism in the West [1, 2]. The most common Extrathyroidal manifestation of the disease is Graves' ophthalmopathy; the diagnosis can be suspected based on clinical findings of the ophthalmopathy, but additional tests are needed. The TSH receptor antibodies also have an essential role in the pathogenesis of ophthalmopathy [1, 3, 4].

Graves' disease is the most common cause of extraocular muscles (EOMs) enlargement, and the main characteristic of Graves' ophthalmopathy is enlarged EOMs [5]. The orbit computed tomography (CT scan) and magnetic resonance imaging (MRI) are essential in the workup of EOMs in Graves 'ophthalmopathy. They are also useful for evaluating disease activity and surgery planning [6, 7]. For diagnosing these cases, the CT scan concomitantly evaluates orbits soft tissues and bones and is also faster and more cost-effective but gives little information about disease activity [8].

Orbit MRI can demonstrate the EOMs edema, especially on turbo inversion recovery magnitude (TIRM) sequence, and differentiates active Graves' ophthalmopathy from inactive cases [9]. Exophthalmos (proptosis) can be measured by Hertel exophthalmometer but has considerable inter-observer variability. The proptosis can be diagnosed and graded on the orbital CT scan and MRI by measuring the vertical line between the posterior corneal surface and the inter-zygomatic line with acceptable accuracy [10, 11].

In this chapter, we discuss the most important clinical aspects of Grave's ophthalmopathy, clinical indications, advantages, and disadvantages, and the most practical findings of the orbit CT scan in these patients to better diagnose and demonstrate the complications of the ophthalmopathy and follow up after appropriate treatment.

2. Graves' disease and ophthalmopathy

The most common extrathyroidal sign of Graves' disease is ophthalmopathy, which is caused by extraocular muscles (EOMs) and orbital fat inflammation due to TSH receptor antibody and cytotoxic T lymphocyte cytokines. Some etiologic factors that can lead to TSH receptor antibodies include environmental, genetic, and intestinal microorganisms. The main environmental factors include vitamin D deficiency, selenium deficiency, smoking, stress, excess uptake of iodine, and viral infections. The genetic factors include the genetic loci such as CD40, MHC, BAFF, and non-coding RNAs as biomarkers for diagnosis and prognosis determination. The intestinal microorganisms' imbalance can also produce cytokines and lead to Graves' disease and ophthalmopathy. These changes mostly lead to Graves' ophthalmopathy signs including proptosis, diplopia, and periorbital edema, which, without treatment, lead to fibrosis of the EOMs which is usually irreversible [12–14]. There are also some risk factors for ophthalmopathy development based on the American Thyroid Association (ATA) 2016. **Table 1** [15]. Smoking is one of the major risk factors, and quitting

Risk factors	Remarks
1. Age	Advanced age: higher risk for severe GO
2. Gender	More frequent in females, more severe in males
3. Genetic	Immunomodulatory genes
4. Anatomic	Wide angle of orbital lateral wall
5. TSHR-Ab	Predicts response to treatment
6. Smoking	Increases progression, decreases treatment response

GO: Grave's ophthalmopathy; TSHR-Ab: thyroid stimulating hormone receptor antibody.

Table 1.
Risk factors of GO.

smoking can prevent development, slow ophthalmopathy progression, and improve the response to treatment [16].

Graves' ophthalmopathy clinical classification is based on the degree of severity and activity of the disease. The clinical severity of the cases is usually evaluated by the European Group on Grave's Orbitopathy (EUGOGO) criteria (**Table 2**), and the clinical activity of ophthalmopathy is usually defined by the clinical activity score (CAS) criteria (**Table 3**) [17–19].

If ophthalmopathy occurs in euthyroid or hypothyroid autoimmune thyroiditis patients, it is called thyroid eye disease (TED). The most common clinical signs of Graves' ophthalmopathy are upper eyelid retraction, periorbital edema with erythema, and proptosis, and the most common finding on computed tomography (CT) scan or magnetic resonance imaging of the orbits is usually enlarged EOMs in both orbits. In clinically unilateral cases, orbital imaging also shows asymmetric bilateral findings. The enlarged EOMs are a common ocular manifestation of Graves' ophthalmopathy. The volumes of enlarged EOM can differentiate active from inactive cases, but still, there are also some controversial results because the EOMs thickening can also be seen in inactive cases [20–22].

In active cases, the EOMs are enlarged and edematous, which can be demonstrated on T2-weighted MRI images of the orbit, but the orbit CT scan is not useful in most cases for differentiating active from inactive Graves' ophthalmopathy because it cannot show the muscles' edema [9].

The EOMs enlargement of Graves' ophthalmopathy is more seen in patients older than 60 years old, and in approximately 40% of the patients, the enlarged EOMs

Mild GO
One or more of the following signs Have a minimum effect on daily life
Mild lid retraction <2 mm
Mild soft tissue involvement
Proptosis <3 mm above normal, considering race and gender (female 18, male 20 mm)
Intermittent diplopia or no diplopia
Lubricants responsive cornea exposure
Moderate-to-severe GO
No sight-threatening GO but needs immunosuppression in active state and surgery in inactive state, two or more following signs
Lid retraction ≥2 mm
Moderate-to-severe soft tissue involvement
Proptosis ≥3 mm above normal, considering race and gender (female 18, male 20 mm)
Constant or inconstant diplopia
Very severe GO
Patients with DON or sight-threatening corneal disorder
Eye subluxation, frozen eye, choroidal folds, and postural visual obscuration

GO: Grave's ophthalmopathy or orbitopathy; EUGOGO: European group on Grave's orbitopathy; DON: dysthyroid optic neuropathy.

Table 2.
Severity of the GO based on the EUGOGO criteria.

CAS in primary exam, *point (1–7)*
1. Spontaneous retrobulbar pain
2. Pain on attempted upward or downward gaze
3. Eyelids swelling
4. Eyelids hyperemia
5. Conjunctival hyperemia
6. Conjunctival swelling (chemosis)
7. Caruncle or plica swelling
Follow-up after 1–3 months, *point (8–10)*
8. Measured proptosis increased >2 mm
9. Decreased eye movement limit of >8° in any direction
10. Decreased visual acuity = 1 Snellen chart line
Active GO = CAS ≥ 3/7 in primary exam or > 4/10 on follow-up *Inactive GO* = CAS < 3/7 in primary exam or ≤ 4/10 on follow-up
GO: Grave's ophthalmopathy.

Table 3.
GO clinical activity score (CAS).

can compress the optic nerve at the orbital apex due to apex crowding and lead to optic neuropathy in 6% of these cases. Orbital fat expansion is more seen in patients younger than 40 years old, although most of the cases have both enlarged EOMs and expanded orbital fat with the predominance of one of them [15, 20, 23]. However, a small number of these patients have only orbital fat expansion without enlarged EOMs, which can lead to proptosis. The orbital fat expansion and EOMs enlargement, the compression of the optic nerve due to enlarged muscles and orbital apex crowding in these patients, and asymmetric proptosis all can be evaluated by the orbit CT scan and MRI, but orbit CT scan can concomitantly evaluate both soft tissues and bones and is also faster and more cost-effective [8, 24–27].

The inferior rectus muscle (IRM) is the most commonly involved EOM in Graves' ophthalmopathy, but the superior rectus muscle (SRM) can be the only muscle involved in 30% of these cases; however, some studies showed that the SRM involvement can be the most commonly involved EOMs in these cases [28–30].

On the other hand, the enlarged SRM has a statistically significant correlation with proptosis, whereas medial rectus muscle (MRM), lateral rectus muscle (LRM), and IRM enlargement do not correlate with proptosis. Superior and inferior oblique muscles can also be involved in Graves' ophthalmopathy and should be evaluated by imaging. In our experience, these muscles are not usually involved, but they are mostly involved in advanced cases. Exophthalmos (proptosis) is commonly measured by Hertel exophthalmometer in clinical settings, and on orbital CT scan or MRI, it is measured based on the length of the arbitrary vertical line between the posterior margin of the eye cornea and the line between both zygomatic bone. (inter-zygomatic line) [10, 31, 32].

The management of Graves' ophthalmopathy consists of immunosuppressive or anti-inflammatory drugs (glucocorticoids), radiation therapy, and rehabilitative surgery. Rehabilitative surgery consists of orbital decompression or corrective surgery for lid retraction or constrictive myopathy and strabismus. The choice of treatment is based on the severity and activity of the ophthalmopathy (**Tables 2** and **3**).

For patients with mild Graves' ophthalmopathy, antithyroid drugs, symptom management, and follow-up are usually done, and in these cases, an orbital CT scan is not usually performed unless there is diplopia or retrobulbar lesion suspicion. In active and moderate-to-severe cases, immuno-suppressive or anti-inflammatory (glucocorticoids) drugs or radiation therapy is the first line of treatment.

In patients with inactive (for at least 6 months) and moderate-to-severe Graves' ophthalmopathy and also for cosmetic purposes, rehabilitative surgery should be considered.

In the case of dysthyroid optic neuropathy (DON) and sight-threatening Graves' ophthalmopathy (very severe ophthalmopathy), first-line treatment is immunosuppressive or anti-inflammatory therapy, and if there is a poor response, emergent rehabilitative surgery is performed [2, 33].

3. Orbital imaging in *Grave's ophthalmopathy*

The diagnosis of Graves' disease is primarily made by laboratory tests for thyroid dysfunction and autoimmunity, but orbital CT scan and MRI have an important role both in the diagnosis and follow-up of Graves' ophthalmopathy cases after appropriate medical and/or surgical management of the disease.

The major advantages of the orbit MRI are no ionizing radiation, optic nerve evaluation, and detection of the active versus inactive (fibrous stage) Graves' ophthalmopathy by demonstrating EOMs edema and signal intensity ratio (SIR) on turbo inversion recovery magnitude (TIRM), short tau inversion recovery (STIR), and T2-weighted sequences. The MRI is not suitable for orbital bone details, it is time-consuming, and it is not a cost-effective imaging modality for these patients [34].

The advantages of the orbit CT scan are great spatial resolution, readily accessible, simultaneous evaluation of the soft tissues and bones of the orbital cavities with acceptable accuracy, cost-effectiveness, and the time-saving imaging modality.

The orbit CT scan also helps evaluate paranasal sinuses, orbital wall remodeling, especially medial orbital walls, EOMs enlargement, and increased orbital fat volume. It is routinely used before orbital decompression surgery and also readily demonstrates post-operative changes. Hence, the orbit CT scan is the preferred imaging modality for diagnosing Graves' ophthalmopathy, and the main purpose of the orbit CT scan in these patients is the evaluation of the degrees of proptosis and EOMs size and density.

The enlarged EOMs provide orbital apex crowding and lead to optic nerve compression, and dysthyroid optic neuropathy (DON). The presence of orbital apex crowding on orbit CT scan images coronal view is strongly correlated with DON in Graves' ophthalmopathy patients and can be estimated by Barrett's muscle index (**Figure 1**) and/or perineural fat effacement by Nugent's method (**Figure 2**) on this view.

A muscle index of ≥67% has a diagnostic sensitivity = 67–70% for compressive DON, and based on Nugent's method, no effacement of the perineural fat is grade 0, 1–25% effacement is grade 1, between 25 and 50% is grade 2, and > 50% effacement is considered as grade 3 [35, 36]. The major disadvantage of the orbit CT scan is that this imaging modality cannot differentiate the active ophthalmopathy from the inactive cases and also has X-ray exposure [8, 9, 29, 37].

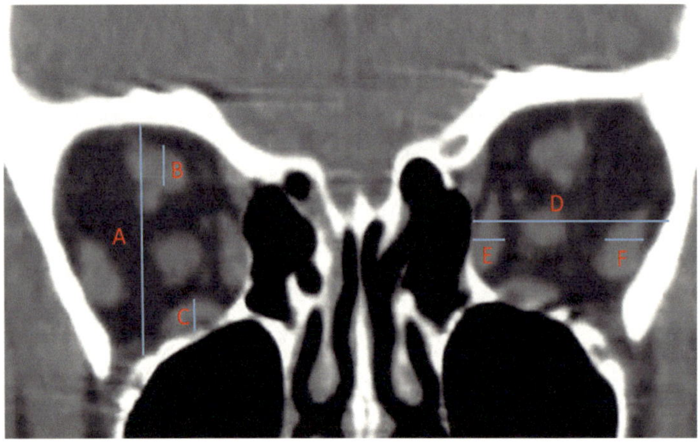

Figure 1.
Orbit CT scan, coronal view. Barret's muscle index: a. The vertical index: B + C/A x 100 b. The horizontal index: E + F/D x 100.

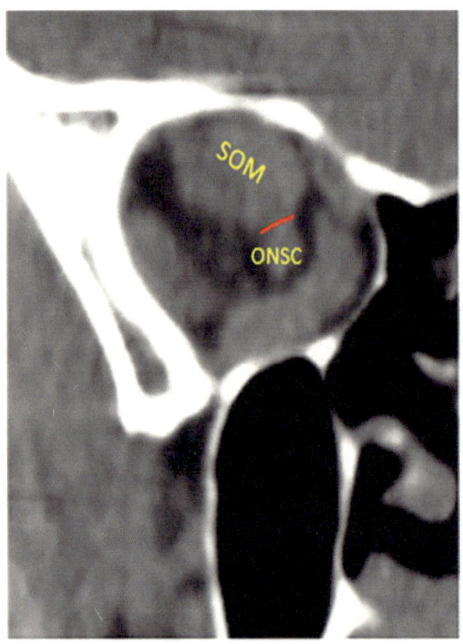

Figure 2.
Orbit CT scan, coronal view. Nugent's method: there is about 25% effacement of the orbital fat (red line) between the optic-nerve-sheath complex (ONSC) and adjacent superior rectus muscle (SOM). Note the remodeling of the orbit medial wall due to the enlarged adjacent medial rectus muscle.

4. Indications and technique of orbit computed tomography (CT) scan

Some important indications of the orbit CT scan include: (1) orbital wall fractures, (2) foreign body detection, (3) Grave's ophthalmopathy evaluation, (4) orbital mass lesion, and (5) orbital inflammatory-infective lesions. Among these indications, the orbit CT scan of Graves' ophthalmopathy patients has noticeable importance from the point of its complications including enlarged EOMs, the severity of proptosis, enlarged orbital at, enlarged lacrimal glands, prolapse of lacrimal glands, orbital apex crowding, DON as previously mentioned [7, 38, 39].

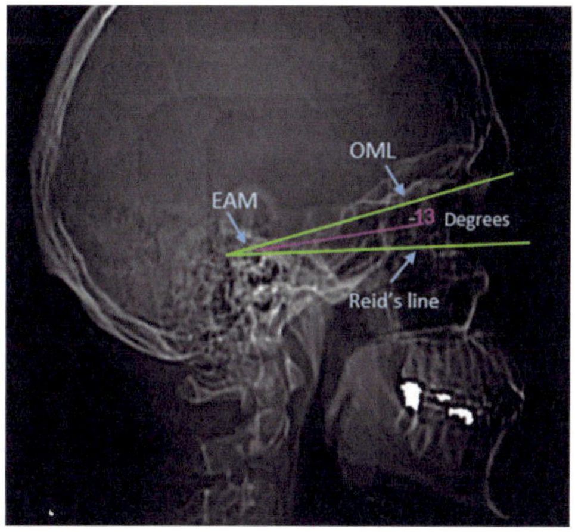

Figure 3.
Lateral skull and face scout view. Localization of reference lines for accurate positioning, and obtaining accurate CT scan slices of the orbital cavities. EAM = external auditory meatus, OML = orbito-meatal line.

In our radiology department, the CT scan machine is the 8-slice Multidetector CT scan (MDCT) GE bright speed. During imaging, the patients lay down in a supine position on the machine table with a head-to-foot orientation, the eyes kept closed, and the gaze of the eyes in a neutral position. In our at least 10 years of experience in the tertiary ophthalmology hospital center, the 8-slice MDCT of the orbit provides appropriate images for demonstrating the details essential for the diagnosis of Graves' ophthalmopathy complications such as orbital apex crowding, EOMs enlargement, proptosis severity, lacrimal glands enlargement and prolapse, and follow-up after appropriate medical and surgical treatments for the hospital orbit subspecialty doctors.

The slices are continuous without gaps, and the thickness of the slice usually equals 1.25–1.50 mm. The Kilovoltage (KV) is 100–120 and the Miliamper X Seconds (MAS) is 80–200, which is usually automatically set up by choosing the appropriate orbit CT scan protocol on the workstation console application. The slices are obtained parallel to Reid's line, which is −10 to −15 degrees to the orbito-meatal line (OML), which is the best reference line for optimally depicting the optic canal. The slices can also be done parallel to OML but are not appropriate for obtaining optimal reconstructed images of the optic canal (**Figure 3**).

Both soft tissue window and bone window on axial view are obtained and reconstructed to coronal and sagittal views by experienced radiology experts through sophisticated applications on the workstation system for better and complementary evaluation of these orbital structures. The intravenous contrast agent injection is not routinely used because it provides no further information unless, on non-contrast images, a mass lesion is suspected. In other words, the iodine within the contrast agents can also exacerbate the clinical symptoms and signs of Graves' ophthalmopathy, and one must be cautious in using the iodine contrast agents in these patients [40, 41].

5. Normal anatomy of the orbit on computed tomography (CT) scan images

The major anatomic contents of the orbits that are readily depicted on orbit CT scan images are eye globes characteristics, eye globes position, extraocular muscles (EOMs) size and shape, the optic nerve-sheath complex (ONSC), orbital fat, lacrimal glands size and position, and the bones of the obits and related paranasal sinuses and all are important anatomic checkpoints in Grave's ophthalmopathy [42, 43].

The eye globe positions can be easily evaluated on orbit CT scan axial images on the section in which the eye lens is seen based on the measurement of the distance between the posterior margin of the eye cornea or posterior sclera of the eye and the inter-zygomatic (IZ) line measured through a vertical line (**Figure 4**). The distance between the anterior margin of the eye's cornea and the IZ line can also be measured, but in our experience, the anterior margin of the cornea cannot be readily seen and/or estimated because of the overlapping of preseptal soft tissues during the orbit CT scan with closed eyes.

The measurement can also be done on the sagittal view in the section where the eye lens is seen. In this view, a line is drawn between the superior and inferior orbital rims that must intersect the lens in people without proptosis, and if the lens is not crossed and located anterior to the line, the proptosis is present. These measurements correlate better with the clinical results of the Hertel exophthalmometer [44–46]. The best view for measuring the size of the EOMs depends on the anatomic location of the muscle (**Figure 5**).

For the superior rectus muscle (SRM) and inferior rectus muscle (IRM), the best view is the coronal section, and for medial rectus muscle (MRM) and lateral rectus muscle (LRM), the best view is the axial section. Superior oblique muscle (SOM) and inferior oblique muscle (IOM) size is measured on axial and coronal views. Both the volume and thickness of the EOMs can be measured [47, 48], but the volume is not readily performed because it is sophisticated and application dependent, and time-consuming; hence, the maximum thickness of the muscles is routinely measured on corresponding and appropriate sections as shown in **Figures 6–8**.

The optic nerve-sheath complex (ONSC) thickness is better measured from the axial view, but the measurement of the complex's volume is not practical, and

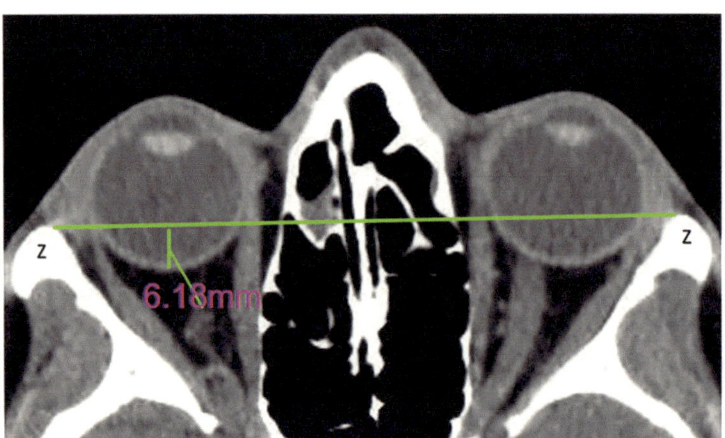

Figure 4.
Evaluation of the proptosis in orbit CT scan, axial view. In normal eye position. At least 5 mm of the eye anterior-posterior (AP) length must be posterior to the inter-zygomatic line if there is less than 5 mm is considered proptosis. Z = Zygoma bone.

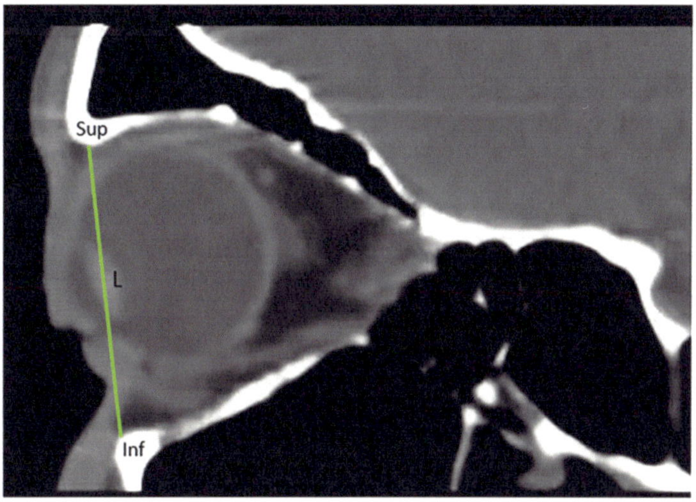

Figure 5.
Evaluation of the proptosis in orbit CT scan, sagittal view. In normal eye position, the line between the superior and inferior orbital rims must intersect the lens. Sup = superior orbital rim, Inf = inferior orbital rim, L = lens.

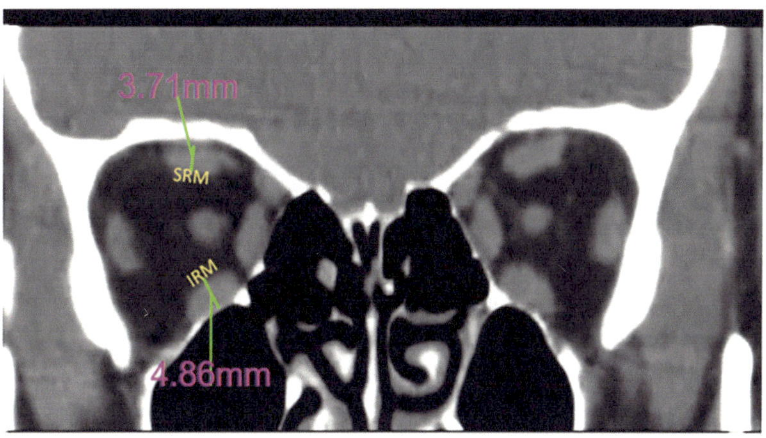

Figure 6.
The measurement of the superior rectus muscle (SRM) and inferior rectus muscle (IRM) thickness in orbit CT scan, coronal view. The SRM and IRM are better seen and measured in the mid-coronal section.

hence, that has not been evaluated in the medical literature so far. The thickness is measured usually on the anterior (retrobulbar), middle, and posterior (adjacent to the optic canal) segments in axial sections. The coronal view also can be used for the ONSC thickness measurement, but it is mainly practical on the mid-section of the complex and the line of measurement must be vertically oriented. On the orbit CT scan images, the subarachnoid space around the optic nerve and the optic nerve body itself cannot be readily separated, therefore, the complex is measured as a whole [45, 49–51]. The retrobulbar segment is usually measured 3 mm posterior to the eye sclera (**Figure 9**).

In our experience, the range of the normal thickness of the extraocular muscles is roughly 3–5 mm, and the normal thickness of intraorbital ONSC in the retrobulbar

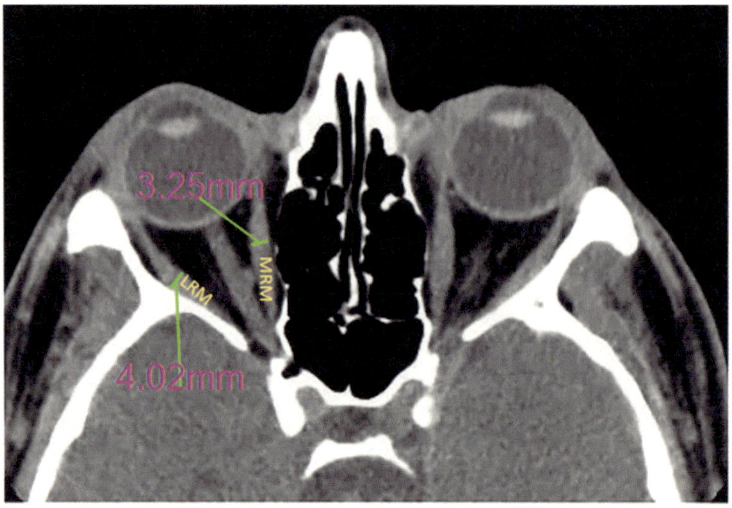

Figure 7.
The measurement of the medial rectus muscle (MRM) and lateral rectus muscle (LRM) thickness in orbit CT scan, axial view. The MRM and LRM are better seen and measured in the mid-axial section.

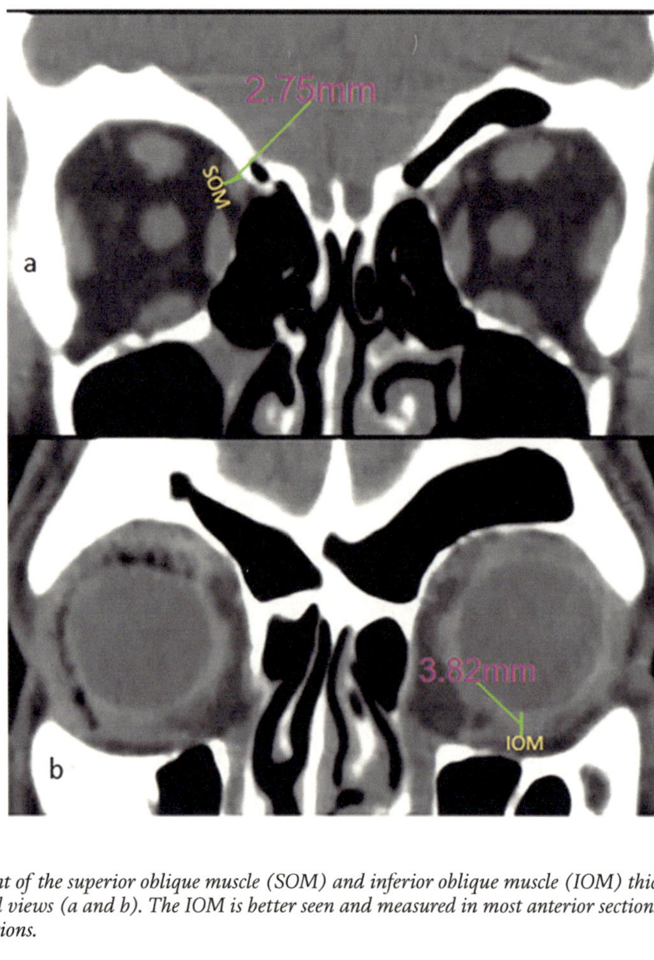

Figure 8.
The measurement of the superior oblique muscle (SOM) and inferior oblique muscle (IOM) thickness in orbit CT scan, coronal views (a and b). The IOM is better seen and measured in most anterior sections and the SOM in mid-coronal sections.

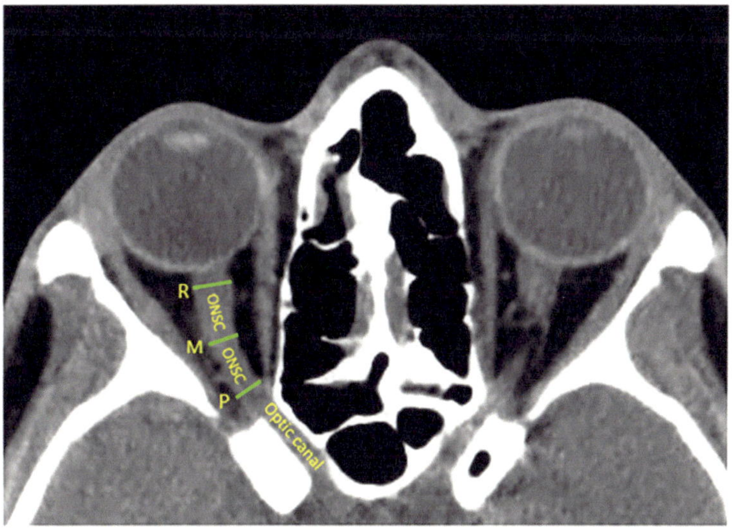

Figure 9.
The measurement of the optic nerve-sheath complex (ONSC) thickness on the retrobulbar (R) 3 mm to the eye posterior sclera, middle (M), and posterior segments (P) adjacent to the optic canal in axial view orbital CT scan.

segment is roughly 4–6 mm, and in the middle segment and segment adjacent to the optic canal is 3–5 mm. Some conducted studies have also included these measurements within these ranges [47, 50–53].

There is no acceptable or practical system for measuring orbital fat linearly, but the volume or cross-sectional area of the orbital fat can be measured, as mentioned in some studies. Fat volume and cross-sectional area measurements are time-consuming, sophisticated, and application-dependent [54–56].

In our experience, whenever there is a protrusion of the orbital fat within the eyelid-orbital fat interface, penetration of the orbital fat within the lacrimal gland-eye sclera interface, MRM tendon-eye sclera interface, and medial canthus-eye sclera interface, the orbital fat can be considered increased in comparison with the clinical exam findings of the orbit and Graves' ophthalmopathy experts [57]. The best view for evaluating the increased orbital fat is on the axial section (**Figure 10**).

The lacrimal glands' size and position are practically measured and evaluated in the section where the major part of the gland is seen (mid-axial section). The size of the lacrimal gland consists of the anterior-posterior (AP) length and transverse (T) width on axial sections, which are commonly increased in Graves' ophthalmopathy and affect the clinical features and surgical results. The volume and/or cross-section of the lacrimal glands can also be measured, but it is time-consuming, sophisticated-application dependent, and not clinically practical. The normal range anterior-posterior (AP) length of the lacrimal gland is usually 15–18 mm, and the normal range of transverse (T) width of the lacrimal gland is usually 5–8 mm [58–60].

Furthermore, in our experience and based on some studies, no more than 50 percent of the AP length of the gland must be located anterior to the inter-zygomatic line on the mid-axial section, and if so, the gland is considered a prolapsed lacrimal gland, which is a major finding in Graves' ophthalmopathy affecting the

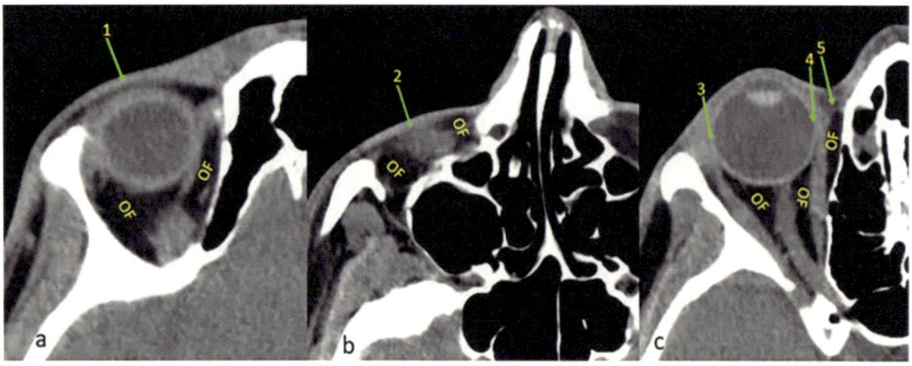

Figure 10.
Orbit CT scan axial sections in different levels in normal individuals. a. upper eyelid level, b. lower eyelid level, and c- lacrimal gland-medial canthus level. 1 = Upper eyelid-orbital fat interface, 2 = Lower eyelid-orbital fat interface, 3 = Lacrimal gland-eye sclera interface, 4 = medial rectus muscle tendon-eye sclera interface, 5 = Medial canthus-eye sclera interface, and OF = orbital fat.

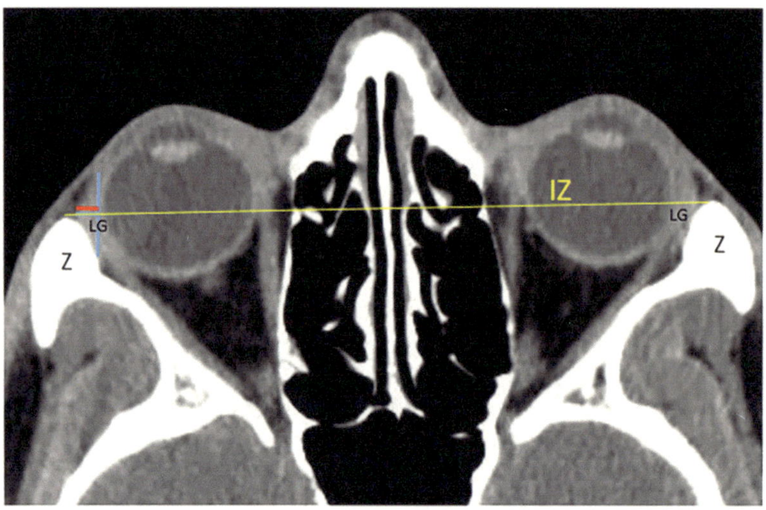

Figure 11.
Lacrimal gland (LG) linear measurement on orbit CT scan mid-axial section. The blue line is the anterior-posterior (AP) length of the gland, the red line is the transverse (T) width of the gland, and the yellow line is inter-zygomatic (IZ). The T width must be perpendicular to the AP length and parallel to the IZ line, and the AP length must be perpendicular to the IZ for accurate measurement of the lacrimal gland size. In normal individuals, no more than 50% of the AP length of the gland must be located anterior to the IZ line. Z = zygoma bones.

clinical features and surgical results (**Figure 11**). Prolapse and/or increased size of the lacrimal glands can have an additive effect on the severity of the proptosis in these patients [61].

The orbit CT scan readily demonstrates the orbital and paranasal sinuses' bony walls shape and modeling and is completely evaluated on axial, coronal, and sagittal sections. The floor of the orbit is best evaluated on the coronal section, the roof on both coronal and sagittal, and the medial and lateral walls on both axial and coronal sections (**Figures 12** and **13**). The orbital apex shape, configuration, and crowding should be evaluated in all three sections [62–64]. CT scan images readily show any

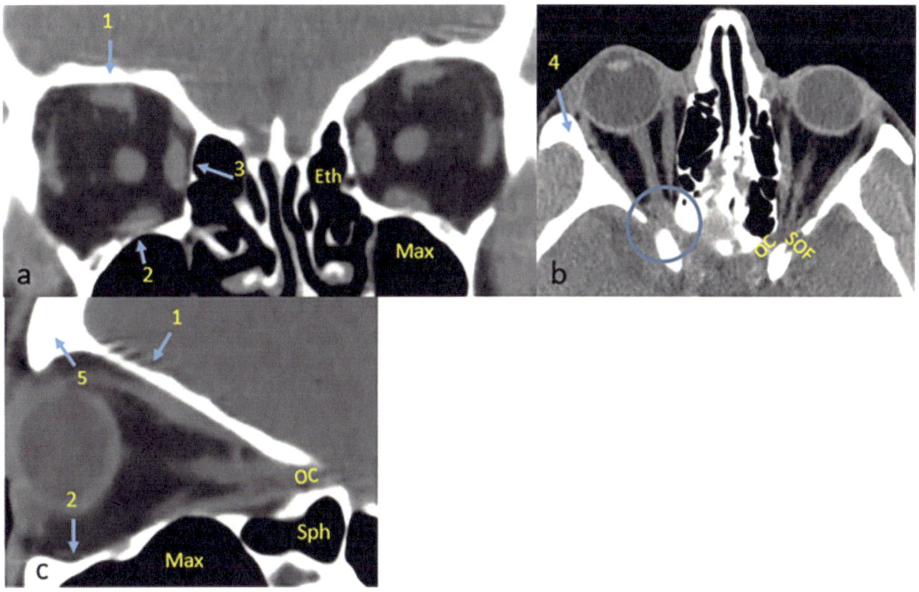

Figure 12.
Orbit CT scan; a-coronal view, b-axial view, and c-sagittal view. 1 = orbital roof, 2 = orbital floor, 3 = orbital medial wall (lamina papyracea), 4 = orbital lateral wall. Eth = ethmoid sinus, Max = maxillary sinus, Sph = sphenoid sinus, OC = optic canal, SOF = superior orbital fissure. Circle on image b = orbital apex.

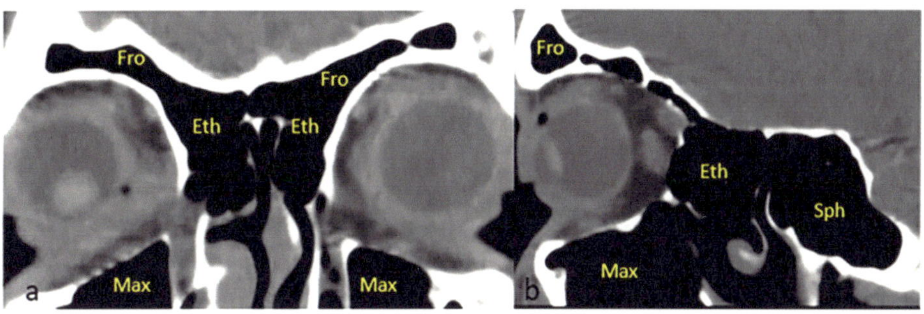

Figure 13.
Orbit CT scan, paranasal sinuses around the orbital cavities: a-coronal view, b-sagittal view. Fro = frontal sinus, Eth = ethmoid sinus, Max = maxillary sinus, Sph = sphenoid sinus.

dehiscence, remodeling, erosion, lytic or sclerotic lesions, and bone changes after decompression surgery (**Figure 14**).

6. Orbit computed tomography (CT) scan in *Grave's ophthalmopathy*

One of the most common complications of Graves' disease is Graves' ophthalmopathy, which can be sight-threatening but can be readily evaluated on the orbit CT scan and/or the orbit magnetic resonance imaging (MRI) based on appropriate orbit CT scan protocol or orbit MRI sequences as previously discussed. The advantage of the CT scan is that it is a more accessible, short-time imaging method, more cost-effective, and also demonstrates both soft tissues and the bones at the same time with clinically

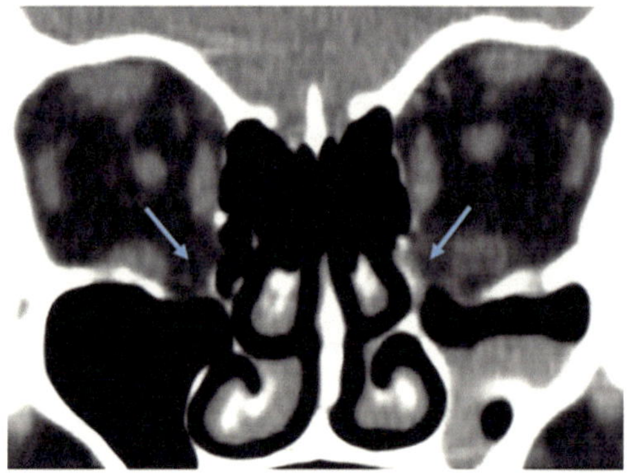

Figure 14.
Orbit CT scan, coronal view. Infero-nasal wall bilateral osteotomy decompression surgery of the GO patient. Arrows.

appropriate resolution. The major disadvantage is that it uses X-rays for imaging, which is harmful to the eye lens, but nowadays, low-dose orbit CT scan protocols solve the problem and increase the safety of the orbit CT scan without decreasing the acceptable resolution of the images in orbital Graves' ophthalmopathy findings [65, 66].

The major defect of the orbit CT scan is that it cannot demonstrate the activity of Graves' ophthalmopathy, and in this situation, the orbit MRI sequences such as Chemical Shift-selective Fat Suppression (CHESS), short inversion time inversion recovery (STIR) do their best, by demonstrating extraocular muscles (EOMs) edema and also measuring the T2 values of the EOMs on T2 weighted sequences for differentiating active from inactive cases and also treatment response control. The orbit MRI can also improve the diagnosis of dysthyroid optic neuropathy (DON), but the orbit CT scan can better predict the risk of DON because of the demonstration of orbital bony structures and orbital apex crowding besides enlarged EOMs [67–69].

Considering the good access, short-time imaging, appropriate resolution, and evaluation of the bones and soft tissues of the orbit at the same time, the orbit CT scan is the most practical and acceptable imaging modality for diagnosis and follow-up of Graves' ophthalmopathy. The major findings on the orbit CT scan of Graves' ophthalmopathy are enlarged extraocular muscles (EOMs), which are the characteristics of these cases, increased orbital fat, proptosis, enlarged lacrimal glands, prolapse of the lacrimal glands, dilated superior ophthalmic veins (SOVs) and orbital apex crowding due to enlarged EOMs which are all readily and accurately seen on CT scan images.

The enlarged EOMs, especially the superior rectus muscle (SRM), correlate with disturbed visual acuity and DON. Based on our experience and some other studies, in Graves' ophthalmopathy, the most commonly involved EOMs are the inferior and medial rectus muscles (IRM and MRM), which are not commonly associated with optic nerve compression and DON. The least commonly involved muscles are the superior and inferior oblique muscles (SOM and IOM). The EOMs can be enlarged without obvious proptosis, and also, proptosis can be due to enlarged orbital fat and not necessarily the enlarged muscles. The younger the patient, the more chance of increased orbital fat; the more advanced the age, the more chance of increased EOMs volume [6, 8, 70, 71]. The enlarged muscles are usually fusiform, and the muscle's tendons are not usually involved (**Figure 15**).

The enlarged EOMs in Graves' ophthalmopathy can have hypodense patches or streaks, which can be due to fatty or lymphocytic infiltration and/or

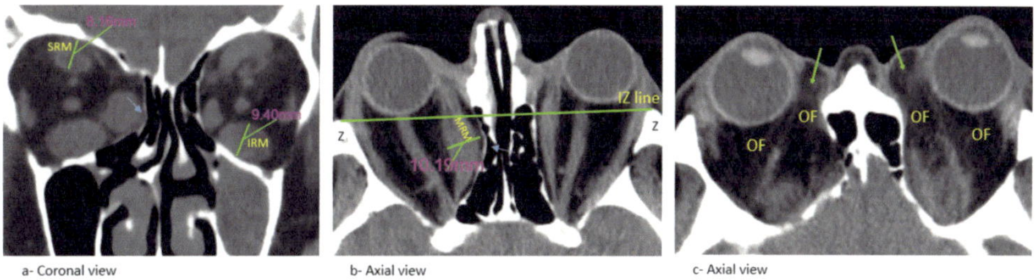

Figure 15.
There are markedly increased EOMs thickness and proptosis (a & b). The eye globes are completely located anterior to the inter-zygomatic line (IZ line) (b). SRM = superior rectus muscle, MRM = medial rectus muscle, IRM = inferior rectus muscle. Notice that the MRM and IRM are larger than other muscles. The arrows point to the deformity of the right orbital medial wall which is due to previous decompression surgery. In this case, there is also increased orbital fat as arrow-pointed in image c with protruded fat within the medial canthus of both sides of the orbital cavities. OF = orbital fat.

mucopolysaccharides accumulation within the muscles, but the mean density of orbital fat is relatively increased [6, 72, 73].

In our experience, decreased density of the EOMs is a specific sign for the diagnosis of Graves' ophthalmopathy. It can readily differentiate the other causes of the enlarged EOMs with fusiform shape and proptosis and also can be seen in these patients without proptosis like some other studies' results (**Figure 16**).

The EOMs are usually enlarged asymmetrically in orbital cavities and can cause pressure remodeling of the bony orbital wall, usually the medial wall (lamina papyracea). The medial orbital wall remodeling is more readily detected in an axial view and can be very similar to the shape of decompression surgery, but clinical history is helpful (**Figure 17**).

In Graves' ophthalmopathy of younger patients, proptosis is mainly caused by only increased orbital fat, and muscles are not enlarged. The fat volume or surface area can be measured in orbit CT scan by some sophisticated applications on workstations but it is time-consuming, cumbersome, and impractical. In our experience, there are some findings on the orbit CT scan images that can demonstrate increased orbital fat content (**Figure 18**).

One of the main clinical and also radiological signs of Graves' ophthalmopathy is prolapse and/or enlargement of lacrimal glands. On orbital CT scan axial view,

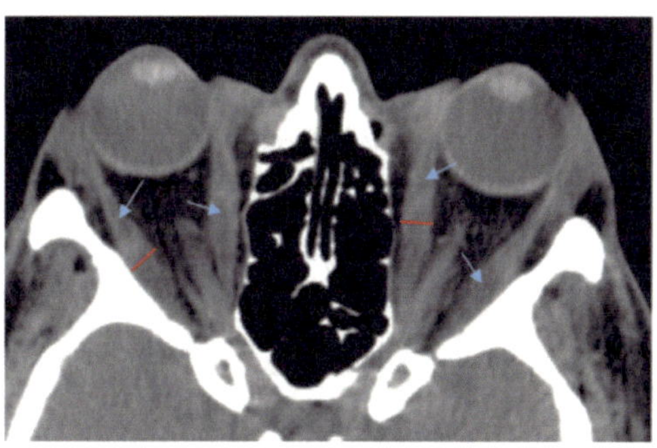

Figure 16.
Orbit CT scan, axial view. There are hypodense linear densities (blue arrows) within the enlarged EOMs (red lines). Note the marked proptosis and also haziness of orbital fat.

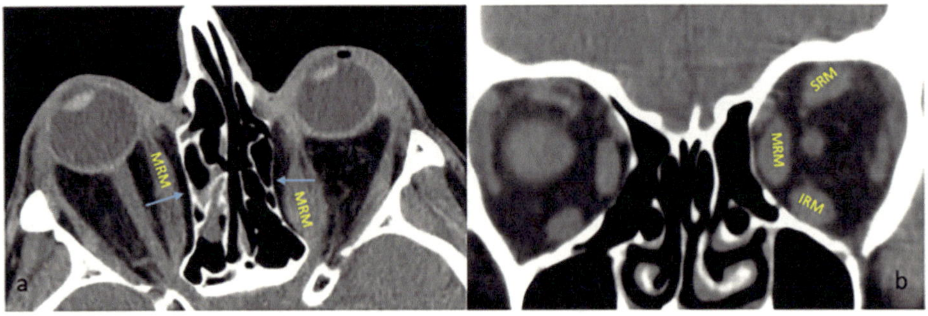

Figure 17.
Orbit CT scan, axial view. a. Remodeling of the medial orbital wall (arrows) due to markedly enlarged medial rectus muscle (MRM) which is more prominent on the left side. Orbit CT scan, coronal view. b. Asymmetric enlargement of the extraocular muscle. Superior, medial, and inferior rectus (SRM, MRM, and IRM) in the left orbit are larger than the right side.

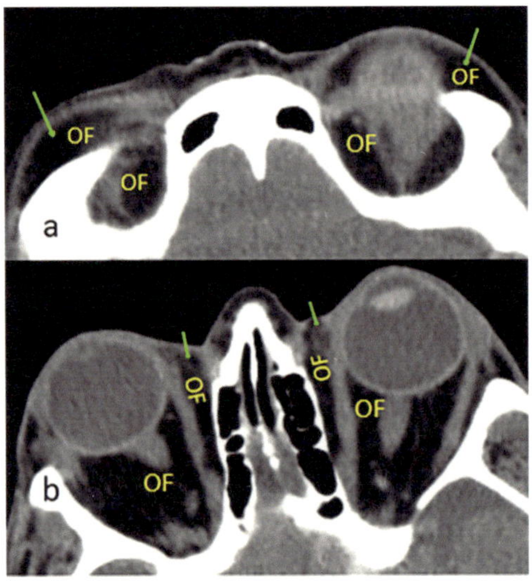

Figure 18.
Orbit CT scan, axial view. a. Demonstrates protruded orbital fat within the upper eyelid subdermal (arrows) b. Demonstrates protruded orbital fat within medial canthus (arrows). As obvious in both images, there is no increased thickness of muscles. OF = orbital fat.

whenever more than 50% of the anterior-posterior length (AP) of the lacrimal glands is located anterior to the inter-zygomatic (IZ) line, prolapse of the gland is considered. The AP length larger than 18 mm and the transverse (T) larger than 8 mm are considered enlarged glands. In chronic advanced cases, fatty-atrophic change also occurs in these glands. The size and location of the lacrimal glands in these patients on orbit CT scan images can predict the severity, progression, and response to treatment in these cases and affect the clinical score of the disease (**Figure 19**) [58, 71, 74].

The superior ophthalmic vein (SOV) is one of the biomarkers in Graves' ophthalmopathy. It can be dilated due to the high flow state of the disease and leads to decreased orbital volume, predisposing the patients to DON, one of the major causes of decreased visual acuity and increased morbidity in these cases, besides the enlarged EOMs and orbital apex crowding. Normal diameter of the SOVs on the orbit CT scan axial view is up to 4–6 mm, and in our experience, measurements

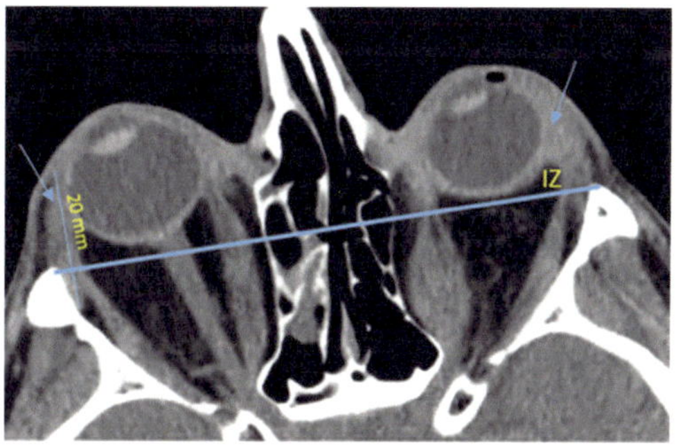

Figure 19.
Orbit CT scan, axial view. The lacrimal glands (arrows) are enlarged (AP length = 20 mm) and more than 50% of the AP length is located anterior to inter-zygomatic line (IZ).

above 6 mm are abnormal SOVs. Orbital apex crowding can also lead to dilated SOVs because of decreased venous outflow [75–77]. The enlarged SOVs can also increase the severity of the proptosis and periorbital edema (**Figure 20**).

The other major sight-threatening complication of Grave's ophthalmopathy is orbital apex crowding due to enlarged EOMs, which is best evaluated in coronal view of orbit CT scan. If there is contact of any of the EOMs border with the optic nerve-sheath complex (ONSC) border in the orbital apex in coronal view (Nugent's method), the risk of the DON can be considered, in other words, the more the effacement of the orbital fat around the ONSC by the enlarged EOMs the more risk of DON.

Based on Nugent's method, no effacement of the perineural fat is grade 0, up to 25% effacement is grade 1, between 25 and 50% is grade 2, and more than 50% effacement is considered as grade 3 (**Figures 2** and **21**) [36, 78].

There is also another criterion (Barrett's index) for predicting the DON based on the severity of the enlargement of the EOMs relative to some dimensions of the orbital cavities. A muscle index ≥67% has a diagnostic sensitivity = 67–70% for compressive DON, as previously mentioned in this chapter (**Figure 22**).

The main indications of rehabilitation-decompression surgery in Grave's ophthalmopathy are moderate-to-severe inactive ophthalmopathy and cases of acute and/or chronic DON with no response to medical treatment. Other indications are

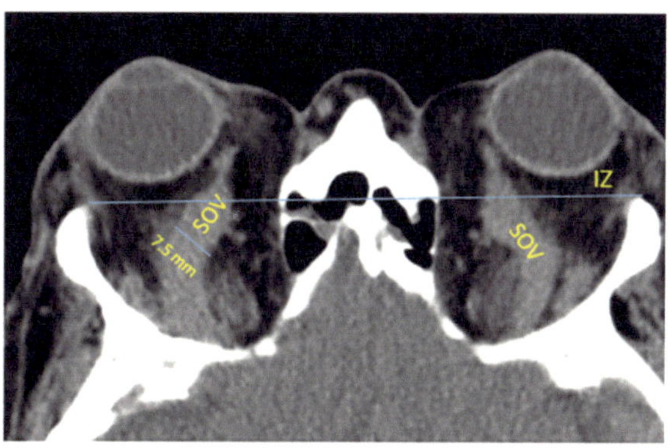

Figure 20.
Obit CT scan, axial view. Markedly distended superior opthalmic vein (SOV) in orbits. Normal diameter is up to 4–6 mm. Note also marked anterior displacement of the eyes relative to the inter-zygomatic (IZ) line.

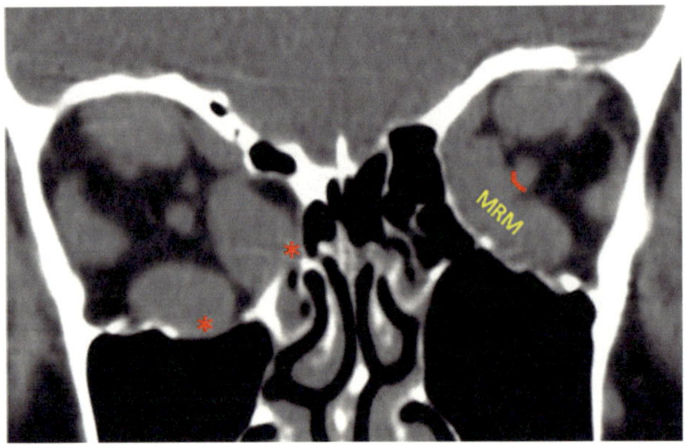

Figure 21.
Orbit CT scan, coronal view. There is the medial-inferior wall osteotomy in the right orbital cavity for expansion of the orbital cavity (asterisks). About 25% of perineural orbital fat effacement (Nugent's method) is due to enlarged medial rectus muscle (MRM) in the left orbit cavity which has not been surgically treated so far (curved line).

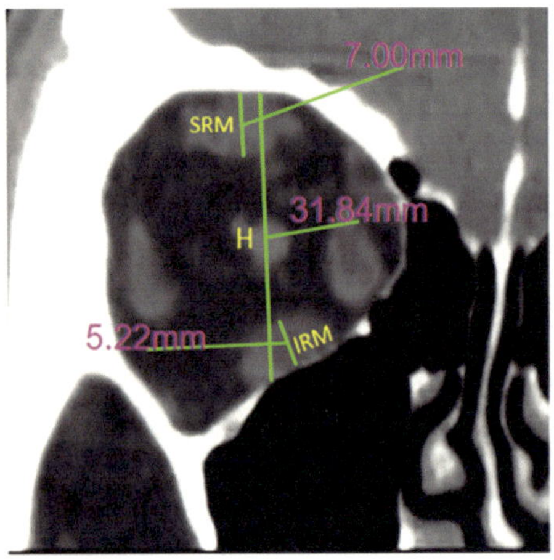

Figure 22.
Obit CT scan, coronal view. The calculated Barret's index = Inferior rectus muscle (IRM) thickness + superior rectus muscle (SRM) thickness/Height of the orbit (H) × 100 = 38% based on this measured thickness in the case.

strabismus repair and lid surgery, which are usually performed after decompression surgery because of the effect of the surgery on the results of the strabismus and lid repair, but these are not the subject of discussion in this chapter.

In Graves' ophthalmopathy, the orbital CT scan is performed preoperatively for evaluation of the severity of the proptosis, extraocular muscles' thickness, orbital fat content, the shape and size of the lacrimal glands, orbital apex crowding, and bony shape and structures of the orbits and adjacent paranasal sinuses.

In addition to clinical exam findings, the above-mentioned biomarkers are evaluated postoperatively and compared with preoperative orbit CT findings of these patients for assessment of the response to treatment.

Decompression surgery can be done on the medial, lateral, and inferior walls of the orbit in isolation or combination and usually decreases the severity of proptosis and improves the visual acuity of the patient, especially in combination [79–82].

The surgery can also be accompanied by orbital fat removal, which can be more effective in decreasing the proptosis severity but has no constant result, and it is case-dependent (**Figure 21**).

7. Conclusion

Graves's disease is an autoimmune disorder of the thyroid gland, and ophthalmopathy is one the most common complications of the disease with major morbidities including sight-threatening dysthyroid optic neuropathy (DON), dysfunctional extraocular muscles leading to strabismus and diplopia, cosmetic problems due to proptosis, periorbital edema and enlarged lacrimal gland with prolapse of the glands. The orbital imaging modalities, the orbit CT scan, and the orbit MRI can be very helpful adjuncts to clinical exams and clinical follow-ups in the prediction and monitoring of the response of ophthalmopathy complications after appropriate medical treatment or decompression surgery. The advantages of the orbit CT scan are cost-effectiveness, ready access, fast imaging, and simultaneous imaging evaluation of both soft tissue and bony orbits, demonstrating orbital apex crowding and predicting the DON, especially before and after decompression surgery for moderate-to-severe inactive cases. The advantages of the orbit MRI are no ionizing radiation, demonstrating activity of the ophthalmopathy based on visible extraocular muscle edema, and measuring the signal intensity ratio (SIR) of the muscles on images of T2-weighted, STIR, and/or TIRM sequences.

Acknowledgements

Dedicated to Ms. "Maryam Afrazi" who gave me the idea and her continuous support helped me with this achievement.

Author details

Shervin Sharifkashani[1,2,3]

1 Tehran University of Medical Sciences, Tehran, Iran

2 Department of Radiology, Farabi Eye Hospital, Tehran, Iran

3 Amir Alam Ear, Nose and Throat (ENT) Hospital, Tehran, Iran

*Address all correspondence to: shervin.sharif.m.d@gmail.com

References

[1] Antonelli A, Fallahi P, Elia G, Ragusa F, Paparo SR, Ruffilli I, et al. Graves' disease: Clinical manifestations, immune pathogenesis (cytokines and chemokines) and therapy. Best Practice and Research Clinical Endocrinology and Metabolism. 2020;**34**(1):101388. DOI: 10.1016/j.beem.2020.101388

[2] Subekti I, Soewondo P, Soebardi S, Darmowidjojo B, Harbuwono DS, Purnamasari D, et al. Practical guidelines management of Graves ophthalmopathy. Acta Medica Indonesiana. 2019;**51**(4)

[3] Ehlers M, Schot M, Allelein S. Graves' disease in clinical perspective. Front Biosci (Landmark Ed). 2019;**24**(1):35-47. DOI: 10.2741/4708

[4] Goichot B, Leenhardt L, Massart C, Raverot V, Tramalloni J, Iraqi H. Diagnostic procedure in suspected Graves' disease. Annales d'Endocrinologie. 2018;**79**(6):608-617. DOI: 10.1016/j.ando.2018.08.002

[5] Smith JT, Hegedust L. Graves' disease. The New England Journal of Medicine. 2016;**375**(16):1552-1565. DOI: 10.1056/NEJMra1510030

[6] Khizar R, Valerie J, Sandy P, Dinesh S. Extraocular muscle enlargement. Graefe's Archive for Clinical and Experimental Ophthalmology. 2022;**260**(11):3419-3435. DOI: 10.1007/s00417-022-05727-1

[7] Luccas R, Rigueto CM, Alves M, Zantut-Wittmann ED, Reis F. Computed tomography, and magnetic resonance imaging approaches to Graves' ophthalmopathy: A narrative review. Frontiers in Endocrinology. 2023;**14**. DOI: 10.3389/fendo.2023.1277961. PMC-PubMed

[8] Pieroni GAC, Gbrim MSE, Monteiro ELR. Imaging studies for diagnosing Graves' orbitopathy and dysthyroid optic neuropathy. Clinics (São Paulo, Brazil). 2012;**67**(11):1327-1334. DOI: 10.6061/clinics/2012 (11)18

[9] Kirsch E, Von Arx G, Hammer B. Imaging in Graves' orbitopathy. Orbit. 2009;**28**(4):219-225. DOI: 10.1080/01676830903047141

[10] Segni M, Bartley BG, Garrity AJ, Bergstralh EJ, Gorman AC. Comparability of proptosis measurements by different techniques. American Journal of Ophthalmology. 2002;**133**(6):813-818. DOI: 10.1016/s0002-9394(02)01429-0

[11] Schmidt P, Kempin R, Langner S, Beule A, Kindler S, Koppe T. Association of anthropometric markers with globe position: A population-based MRI study. Plos One. 7 Feb 2019;**14**(2):e0211817. DOI: 10.1371/journal.pone.0211817. PMC-PubMed

[12] Lane LC, Louise WC, Cheetham T. Graves' disease: Moving forwards. Archives of Disease in Childhood. 2023;**108**:276-282. DOI: 10.1136/archdischild-2022-323905

[13] Smith TJ. Pathogenesis of Graves' orbitopathy: A 2010 update. Journal of Endocrinological Investigation. 2010;**33**(6):414-421. DOI: 10.1007/BF03346614

[14] Li Z, Cestari MD, Fortin E. Thyroid eye disease: What is new to know? Current Opinion in Ophthalmology. 2018;**29**(6):528-534. DOI: 10.1097/ICU.0000000000000529

[15] Ross SD, Burch BH, Cooper SD, Greenlee MC, Laurberg P, Maia AL,

et al. American thyroid association guidelines for diagnosis and management of hyperthyroidism and other causes of thyrotoxicosis. Thyroid. 2016, 2016;**26**(10):1343-1421. DOI: 10.1089/thy.2016.0229

[16] Thornton J, Kelly SP, Harrison RA, Edwards R. Cigarette smoking and thyroid eye disease: A systematic review. Eye. 2007;**21**:1135-1145. DOI: 10.1038/sj.eye.6702603

[17] Bartalena L, Baldesch L, Boboridis K, Eckstein A, Kahaly JG, Marcocci C, et al. The 2016 European thyroid association/European group on Grave's orbitopathy guidelines for the management of Graves' orbitopathy. European Thyroid Journal. 2016;**5**(1):9-26. DOI: 10.1159/000443828

[18] Bartalena L, Kahaly GJ, Baldeschi L, Dayan CM, Eckstein A, Marcocci C, et al. The 2021 European group on Graves orbitopathy (EUGOGO) clinical practice guidelines for the medical management of Graves' orbitopathy. European Journal of Endocrinology. 2021;**185**(4):G43-G67. DOI: 10.1530/EJE-21-0479

[19] Bartalena L, Baldeschi L, Dickinson JA, Eckstein A, Kendall-Taylor P, Marcocci C, et al. Consensus statement of the European group on Grave's orbitopathy (EUGOGO) on the management of Graves' orbitopathy. Thyroid. 2008;**18**(3):333-346. DOI: 10.1089/thy.2007.0315

[20] Bahn SR. Graves' ophthalmopathy. The New England Journal of Medicine. 2010;**362**(8):726-738. DOI: 10.1056/NEJMra0905750

[21] Byun JS, Moon NJ, Lee JK. Quantitative analysis of orbital soft tissues on computed tomography to assess the activity of thyroid-associated orbitopathy. Graefe's Archive for Clinical and Experimental Ophthalmology. 2017;**255**(2):413-420. DOI: 10.1007/s00417-016-3538-0

[22] Politi LS, Godi C, Cammarata G, Ambrosi A, Ladanza A, Lanzi R, et al. Magnetic resonance imaging with diffusion-weighted imaging in the evaluation of thyroid-associated orbitopathy: Getting below the tip of the iceberg. European Radiology. 2014;**24**(5):1118-1126. DOI: 10.1007/s00330-014-3103-3

[23] Dolman JP. Evaluating Graves' orbitopathy, Best Practice and Research. Clinical Endocrinology and Metabolism. 2012;**26**(3):229-248. DOI: 10.1016/j.beem.2011.11.007

[24] Bartley GB. The epidemiologic characteristics and clinical course of ophthalmopathy associated with autoimmune thyroid disease in Olmsted County, Minnesota. Transactions of the American Ophthalmological Society. 1994;**92**:477-588

[25] Regensburg IN, Wiersinga MW, Berendschot Tos TJM, Potgieser P, Mourits PM. Do subtypes of graves' orbitopathy exist? Ophthalmology. 2011;**118**(1):191-196. DOI: 10.1016/j.ophtha.2010.04.004

[26] Lo C, Ugradar S, Rootman D. Management of graves myopathy, orbital imaging in thyroid-related orbitopathy. Journal of AAPOS. 2018;**22**(4):256.e1-256.e256256. DOI: 10.1016/j.jaapos.2018.06.002

[27] Wémeau J-L, Klein M, Sadoul JL, Briet C, Vélayoudom-Céphise F-L. Graves' disease: Introduction, epidemiology, endogenous and environmental pathogenic factors. Annales d'endocrinologie. 2018;**79**(6):599-607. DOI: 10.1016/j.ando.2018.09.002

[28] Feldon SE, Weiner JM. Clinical significance of extraocular muscle volumes in Graves' ophthalmopathy: A quantitative computed tomography study. Archives of Ophthalmology. 1982;**100**(8):1266-1269. DOI: 10.1001/archopht.1982.01030040244006

[29] Starks SV, Reinshagen LK, Lee GN, Freitag KS. Visual field and orbital computed tomography correlation in dysthyroid optic neuropathy due to thyroid eye disease. Orbit. 2020;**39**(2):77-83. DOI: 10.1080/01676830.2019.1600150

[30] Wang Y, Mettu P, Broadbent T, Radke P, Firl K, Shepherd JB, et al. Thyroid eye disease presenting with superior rectus/levator complex enlargement. Orbit. 2020;**39**(1):5-12. DOI: 10.1080/01676830.2019.1594969

[31] Hudson HL, Levin L, Feldon SE. Grave's exophthalmos unrelated to extraocular muscle enlargement. Superior Rectus Muscle Inflammation May Induce Venous Obstruction, Ophthalmology. 1991;**98**(10):1495-1499. DOI: 10.1016/s0161-6420(91)32099-2

[32] Kakizaki H, Zako M, Masayoshi I. Thyroid-associated inferior oblique myopathy. Ophthalmology. 2007;**114**(11):2106. DOI: 10.1016/j.ophtha.2007.04.034

[33] San MI, Arenas M, Carmona R, Rutllan J, Medina-Rivero F, Lara P. Review of the treatment of Graves' ophthalmopathy: The role of the new radiation techniques. Saudi Journal of Ophthalmology. 2018;**32**(2):139-145. DOI: 10.1016/j.sjopt.2017.09.003

[34] Rodríguez-González N, Pérez-Rico C, López-Para GR, Arévalo-Serrano J, Del Amo García B, Calzada DL, et al. Short-tau inversion-recovery (STIR) sequence magnetic resonance imaging evaluation of orbital structures in Graves' orbitopathy. Archivos de la Sociedad Española de Oftalmología. 2011;**86**(11):351-357. DOI: 10.1016/j.oftal.2011.06.010

[35] Barrett L, Glatt HJ, Burde RM, Gado MH. Optic nerve dysfunction in thyroid eye disease: CT. Radiology. 1988;**167**(2):503-507. DOI: 10.1148/radiology.167.2.3357962

[36] Nugent RA, Belkin RI, Neigel JM, Rootman J, Robertson WD, Spinelli J, et al. Graves orbitopathy: Correlation of CT and clinical findings. Radiology. 1990;**177**(3):675-682. DOI: 10.1148/radiology.177.3.2243967

[37] Ochmann A, Winder M, Nalewajka-Kołodziejczak J, Chudek J. Current imaging methods for assessing graves' orbitopathy activity with particular emphasis on FDG-PET. Frontiers in Endocrinology (Lausanne). 2023;**14**:1138569. DOI: 10.3389/fendo.2023.1138569.eCollection 2023

[38] Wu YA, Jebodhsingh K, Le T, Law C, Tucker AN, Deangelis D, et al. Indications for orbital imaging by the oculoplastic surgeon. Ophthalmic Plastic and Reconstructive Surgery. 2011;**27**(4):260-262. DOI: 10.1097/IOP.0b013e31820b0365

[39] Ferreira AT, Saraiva P, Genders SW, Buchem MV, Luyten GPM, Beenakker J-W. CT and MR imaging of orbital inflammation. Neuroradiology. 2018;**60**(12):1253-1266. DOI: 10.1007/s00234-018-2103-4

[40] Citrin CM. High-resolution orbital computed tomography. Journal of Computer Assisted Tomography. 1986;**10**(5):810-816. DOI: 10.1097/00004728-198609000-00019

[41] Beck TJ, Rosenbaum AE, Miller NR. Orbital computed tomography:

Technical aspects. International Ophthalmology Clinics. 1982;**22**(4):7-43. DOI: 10.1097/00004397-198202240-00004

[42] Sas TN, Camen GC, Stefanescu A, Gheonea A I. Imaging evaluation of the orbit in Graves ophthalmopathy. Current Health Sciences Journal. 2015;**41**(3):285-287. DOI: 10.12865/CHSJ.41.03.16

[43] Tawfik AH, Abdelhalim A, Elkafrawy HM. Computed tomography of the orbit - A review and an update. Saudi Journal of Ophthalmology. 2012;**26**(4):409-418. DOI: 10.1016/j.sjopt.2012.07.004

[44] Park NR, Moon JH, Lee JK. Hertel exophthalmometer versus computed tomography scan in proptosis estimation in thyroid-associated orbitopathy. Clinical Ophthalmology. 2019;**13**:1461-1467. DOI: 10.2147/OPTH.S216838. eCollection 2019

[45] Gupta V, Prabhakar A, Yadav M, Khandelwal N. Computed tomography imaging-based normative orbital measurement in Indian population. Indian Journal of Ophthalmology. 2019;**67**(5):659-663. DOI: 10.4103/ijo.IJO_1187_18

[46] Melki I, Nassej O, Maroua E, Amal B, Bouzaidi K. Radiological Aspects of Proptosis, Educational Exhibit, ECR 2017/C-0990. 2017. DOI: 10.1594/ecr2017/C-0990

[47] Zhang Z-H, Chen Y, Wang Y, Meng W, Fang H-Y, Xu D-D, et al. Normative measurements of extraocular musculature by multislice computed tomography. Chinese Medical Sciences Journal. 2013;**27**(4):232-236. DOI: 10.1016/s1001-9294(13)60007-3

[48] Lee J-Y, Bae K, Park K-A, Lyu IJ, Oh SY. Correlation between extraocular muscle size measured by computed tomography and the vertical angle of deviation in thyroid eye disease. Plus One. 28 Jan 2016;**11**(1):e0148167. DOI: 10.1371/journal.pone.0148167. PMC-PubMed

[49] Evereklioglu C, Sevim DG, Horozoglu F, Polat AO, Sener H, Coskun A, et al. Computed tomographic thickness of retrobulbar optic nerve is decreased in glaucoma patients and is negatively correlated with disease severity. Cureus. 2022;**14**(11):e31066. DOI: 10.7759/cureus.31066.eCollection 2022 Nov

[50] Vaiman M, Abuita R, Bekerman I. Optic nerve sheath diameters in healthy adults measured by computer tomography. International Journal of Ophthalmology. 2015;**8**(6):1240-1244. DOI: 10.3980/j.issn.2222-3959.2015.06.30.eCollection 2015

[51] Ominde SB, Abadom EG, Ikubor EJ, Achapu CL, Enakpoya OP, Igbigbi SP. Normal diameter of the optic nerve using magnetic resonance imaging: A retrospective Nigerian study. Saudi Journal of Ophthalmology. 2024;**38**(1):53-58. DOI: 10.4103/sjopt.sjopt_189_23.eCollection 2024 Jan-Mar

[52] Ozgen A, Ariyurek M. Normative measurements of orbital structures using CT. AJR. American Journal of Roentgenology. 1998;**170**(4):1093-1096. DOI: 10.2214/ajr.170.4.9530066

[53] Akturk Y, Simsir BD, Hekimoğlu B. Measurement of optic nerve sheath diameter by computed tomography in the pediatric population: Normal values. Journal of Pediatric Ophthalmology and Strabismus. 2024;**61**(1):38-43. DOI: 10.3928/01913913-20230331-02

[54] Kaichi Y, Tanitame K, Terada H, Itakura H, Ohno H, Yoneda M, et al.

Thyroid-associated orbitopathy: Quantitative evaluation of the orbital fat volume and edema using IDEAL-FSE. European Journal of Radialogy Open. 2019;**6**:182-186. DOI: 10.1016/j.ejro.2019.05.003

[55] Kim HC, Yoon SW, Lew H. Usefulness of the ratio of orbital fat to total orbit area in mild-to-moderate thyroid-associated ophthalmopathy. The British Journal of Radiology. 2015;**88**(1053):20150164. DOI: 10.1259/bjr.20150164

[56] Forbes G, Gorman CA, Brennan MD, Gehring DG, Ilstrup DM, Earnest F. Ophthalmopathy of Graves' disease: Computerized volume measurements of the orbital fat and muscle. AJNR. American Journal of Neuroradiology. 1986;**7**(4):651-656

[57] Seedat A, Seedat S, Moosa EIS. Proptosis with increased orbital fat in an obese patient. Case Reports in Radiology. 2020. DOI: 10.1155/2020/8832704

[58] Caltabiano C, Rana KB, Beecher M, Selva D. Radiological measurements of the lacrimal gland in thyroid eye disease. International Ophthalmology. 2024;**44**:11. DOI: 10.1007/s10792-024-02991-4

[59] Lee JS, Lee H, Kim JW, Chang M, Park M, Baek S. Computed tomographic dimensions of the lacrimal gland in healthy orbits. The Journal of Craniofacial Surgery. 2013;**24**(3):712-715. DOI: 10.1097/SCS.0b013e31827fecc0

[60] Nawaz S, Lal S, Butt R, Ali M, Shahani B, Dadlani A. Computed tomography evaluation of normal lacrimal gland dimensions in the adult Pakistani population. Cureus. 24 Mar 2020;**12**(3):e7393. DOI: 10.7759/cureus.7393. PMC-PubMed

[61] Gao Y, Chang Q, Li Y, Zhang H, Hou Z, Zhang Z, et al. Correlation between extent of lacrimal gland prolapse and clinical features of thyroid-associated ophthalmopathy: A retrospective observational study. BMC Ophthalmology. 2022;**22**(66). DOI: 10.1186/s12886-022-02270-9. PMC-PubMed

[62] Kaya M, Cankal F, Tekdemir I. Bone dehiscences of medial orbital wall on computed tomography and assessment of terminological errors in literature. Folia Morphologica. 2022;**81**(1):175-182. DOI: 10.5603/FM.a2021.0004

[63] Chan L-L, Tan H-E, Fook-Chong S, Teo T-H, Lim L-H, Seah L-L. Graves ophthalmopathy: The bony orbit in optic neuropathy, its apical angular capacity, and impact on prediction of risk. American Journal of Neuroradiology. 2009;**30**(3):597-602. DOI: 10.3174/ajnr.A1413

[64] Albano de Guimarães J, Chahud F, Santos BG, Cruz EA, Velasco A. Computed tomography and magnetic resonance imaging of an unusual intraconal orbital osteoma. Orbit. 2023;**42**(3):343-346. DOI: 10.1080/01676830.2021.2012206

[65] Lee H-J, Kim J, Kim KW, Lee S-K, Yoon JS. Feasibility of a low-dose orbital CT protocol with a knowledge-based iterative model reconstruction algorithm for evaluating Graves' orbitopathy. Clinical Imaging. 2018;**51**:327-331. DOI: 10.1016/j.clinimag.2018.06.018

[66] Duarte ML, Dos Santos LR, Bulle OAS, Iared W, Peccin MS. Computed tomography with low-dose radiation versus standard-dose radiation for diagnosing fractures: Systematic review and meta-analysis. São Paulo Medical Journal. 2021;**139**(4):388-397. DOI: 10.1590/1516-3180.2020.0374.R3.1902021

[67] Song C, Luo Y, Yu G, Chen H, Shen J. Current insights of applying MRI in Graves' ophthalmopathy. Frontiers in Endocrinology (Lausanne). 2022;**13**:991588. DOI: 10.3389/fendo.2022.991588

[68] Cheng J, Zhang X, Lian J, Piao Z, Zhou L, Gou X, et al. Evaluation of activity of Graves' orbitopathy with multiparameter orbital magnetic resonance imaging (MRI). Quantitative Imaging in Medicine and Surgery. 2023;**13**(5):3040-3049. DOI: 10.21037/qims-22-814

[69] Cheng S, Ming Y, Hu M, Zhang Y, Jiang F, Wang XI et al. Risk prediction of dysthyroid optic neuropathy based on CT imaging features combined the bony orbit with the soft tissue structures, Frontiers in Medicine (Lausanne). 2022;**9**:936819. DOI:10.3389/fmed.2022.936819.eCollection2022

[70] Chaganti S, Mundy K, DeLisi PM, Nelson MK, Harrigan LR, Galloway LR, et al. Assessment of orbital computed tomography (CT) imaging biomarkers in patients with thyroid eye disease. Journal of Digital Imaging. 2019;**32**(6):987-994. DOI: 10.1007/s10278-019-00195-2

[71] Wiersinga M, Regensburg IN, Mourits PM. Differential involvement of orbital fat and extraocular muscles in graves' ophthalmopathy. European Thyroid Journal. 2013;**2**(1):14-21. DOI: 10.1159/000348246

[72] Hutchings RK, Fritzhand JS, Esmaeli B, Koka K, Zhao J, Ahmed S, et al. Graves' eye disease: Clinical and radiological diagnosis. Biomedicine. 2023;**11**(2):312. DOI: 10.3390/biomedicines11020312

[73] Regensburg IN, Wiersinga MW, Berendschot Tos TJM, Saeed P, Mourits PM. Densities of orbital fat and extraocular muscles in graves orbitopathy patients and controls. Ophthalmic Plastic & Reconstructive Surgery. 2011;**27**(4):236-240. DOI: 10.1097/IOP.0b013e31820365d5

[74] Starčević A, Radojičić Z, Stefanović AD, Trivić A, Milić I, Milić M, et al. Morphometric and volumetric analysis of lacrimal glands in patients with thyroid eye disease. Scientific Reports. 2023;**13**(16345). DOI: 10.1038/s41598-023-43083-0. PMC-PubMed

[75] Yu B, Gong C, Ji Y-F, Xia Y, Tu Y-H, Wu W-C. Predictive parameters on CT scan for dysthyroid optic neuropathy. International Journal of Ophthalmology. 2020;**13**(8):1266-1271. DOI:10.18240/ijo.2020.08.13

[76] Lima BDR, Perry DJ. Superior ophthalmic vein enlargement and increased muscle index in dysthyroid optic neuropathy, ophthalmic. Plastic and Reconstructive Surgery. 2013;**29**(3):147-149. DOI: 10.1097/IOP.0b013e3182831bd8

[77] Monteiro LRM, Moritz BSR, Neto HA, Benabou EJ. Color Doppler imaging of the superior ophthalmic vein in patients with Graves' orbitopathy before and after treatment of congestive disease. Clinics (São Paulo, Brazil). 2011;**66**(8):1329-1334. DOI: 10.1590/s1807-59322011000800004

[78] Gonçalves ACP, Silva LN, Gebrim EMMS, Monteiro MLR. Quantification of orbital apex crowding for screening of dysthyroid optic neuropathy using multidetector CT. American Journal of Neuroradiology. Sep 2012;**33**(8):1602-1607. DOI: 10.3174/ajnr.A3029

[79] Shorr N, Seiff SR. The four stages of surgical rehabilitation of the patient with dysthyroid ophthalmopathy.

Ophthalmology. 1986;**93**:476-483. DOI: 10.1016/s0161-6420(86)33712-6

[80] Naik MN, Nair AG, Gupta A, Kamal S. Minimally invasive surgery for thyroid eye disease. Indian Journal of Ophthalmology. 2015;**63**:847-853. DOI: 10.4103/0301-4738.171967

[81] Cubuk MO, Konuk O, Unal M. Orbital decompression surgery for the treatment of Graves' ophthalmopathy: Comparison of different techniques and long-term results. International Journal of Ophthalmology. 2018;**11**(8):1363-1370. DOI: 10.18240/ijo.2018.08.18

[82] Braun LT, Bhadkamkar AM, Kevin JT, Weber CA, Marx PD. Orbital decompression for thyroid eye disease. Seminars in Plastic Surgery. 2017;**31**(1):40-45. DOI: 10.1055/s-0037-1598192

Section 3

Graves' Disease Treatment

Chapter 5

Graves' Disease: From Pathophysiology to Novel Therapeutic Aspects

Ifigenia Kostoglou-Athanassiou, Lambros Athanassiou and Panagiotis Athanassiou

Abstract

Hyperthyroidism is characterized by increased levels of thyroid hormones in the blood which are secreted either from the thyroid or from other sources. It is a common thyroid disorder which may be due to various causes. It may be of an autoimmune etiology or may be due to autonomous secretion of thyroid hormones from autonomous or toxic thyroid adenomas or to inflammation which causes destruction of thyroid parenchyma, and finally from production of thyroid hormones from other sources than the thyroid such as ectopic thyroid tissue in the ovaries or from excessive intake of thyroid hormones. Patient history as well as clinical signs, which may be weight loss, tachycardia, rarely atrial fibrillation, fatigue, muscle weakness and very rarely periodic paralysis, increased perspiration, gastrointestinal and neuropsychiatric symptoms, goiter and other symptoms. Graves' disease is characterized by hyperthyroidism and extrathyroidal manifestations, such as ophthalmopathy and pretibial myxedema. Laboratory investigations include measurement of thyroid hormones in the blood, where T_3 and T_4 are increased and thyroid-stimulating hormone (TSH) decreased. Both T and B lymphocytes are involved in the pathogenesis of Graves' disease. Antithyroid drugs, radioiodine, thyroidectomy and novel biological agents are used in the treatment of the disease.

Keywords: hyperthyroidism, Graves' disease, toxic multinodular goiter, toxic adenoma, thyroiditis, thyroid ophthalmopathy, pretibial myxedema

1. Introduction

Hyperthyroidism is a syndrome which is due to exposure of body tissues to excessive concentrations of thyroid hormones, T_3 and T_4 in the blood. The most common causes are Graves' disease, toxic multinodular goiter, toxic adenoma and various forms of thyroiditis. Hyperthyroidism may be due to excessive thyroxine administration in various thyroid diseases. Disease severity may vary depending on the level of thyroid hormones, and it may be classified as subclinical hyperthyroidism, clinical hyperthyroidism or thyrotoxic crisis. Clinical findings depend on disease severity, patient age, presence or absence of extrathyroidal manifestations and disease cause.

Unusual forms of hyperthyroidism are those due to extrathyroidal sources of thyroid hormone secretion, such as a pituitary adenoma which secretes TSH, resistance to thyroid hormones, or trophoblastic tumors. In this case, the cause may evade diagnosis and patients may not get the proper treatment promptly. Knowledge of the causes of hyperthyroidism may lead to proper diagnosis and treatment. Hyperthyroidism treatment depends on the cause of the disease and varies from follow-up to conservative treatment to surgery.

Hyperthyroidism is a disease which may interest physicians of various specialties such as endocrinologists, internists, cardiologists, obstetricians and gynecologists.

Various causes of hyperthyroidism exist. The diagnosis of the cause of hyperthyroidism is important, as natural history and treatment depend on the cause of the disease. The cause may be diagnosed from history and clinical examination. Important findings are symptom duration, thyroid enlargement, the presence of thyroid nodules in palpation or on ultrasonography, pain in the area of the thyroid on palpation and the presence of extrathyroidal manifestations in Graves' disease. Thyroid hormone and antibodies measurement, thyroid ultrasonography and scintigraphy are necessary and assist in the diagnosis.

2. Graves' disease

Graves' disease is the commonest form of hyperthyroidism worldwide. Hyperthyroidism is characterized by a prevalence of 1.2% worldwide, 0.5% clinical and 0.7% subclinical hyperthyroidism [1]. Graves' disease is the cause of hyperthyroidism in a percentage of 60–80% of cases of hyperthyroidism [2]. Graves' disease is more prevalent in female patients as compared to male patients by a ratio of 7 to 10:1. However, Graves' disease may be more severe in male patients.

Graves' disease is an autoimmune disease. Antibodies against TSH receptors (TRAbs) stimulate the receptors, activate adenylate cyclase and increase the production of thyroid hormones, increase thyroid size and thyroid vascularization. Etiology is thought to be related to genetic susceptibility and the effect of environmental factors or endogenous factors [3].

Clinical findings are related to multiple organ systems. In the thyroid goiter may be observed. Ocular symptoms include proptosis, erythema of the conjunctiva and others. Skin manifestations include pretibial myxedema and acropathy.

Ocular manifestations are attributed to infiltration of the ocular apparatus by immune cells. It is an autoimmune disorder. Antibodies against the TSH receptor are thought to target retrobulbar tissues and activate invasion by T lymphocytes. TSH receptor is conjugated with a G protein which is detected in the surface of epithelial thyroid cells. TSH is bound to its receptor and regulates thyroid growth and synthesis and secretion of thyroid hormones. TSH receptor is the major autoantigen in Graves' disease and it is the target of T lymphocytes and autoantibodies which either stimulate the thyroid gland and lead to hyperthyroidism or block endogenous TSH, ultimately leading to hypothyroidism. Fibroblasts are stimulated by cytokines and produce glycosaminoglycans which induce the development of ophthalmopathy in 20–40% of patients with Graves' disease [4–6]. Symptoms are usually mild with minimal pain, tear flow, sensation of a foreign body within the eye and photophobia. In a proportion of 3–5% symptoms may be severe with intense pain, diplopia and loss of vision. Ophthalmopathy may also exist without hyperthyroidism in 10% of Graves' disease patients. In most patients, ophthalmopathy affects both eyes; however, in some cases, it may affect only one eye [7, 8].

Myxedema in Graves' disease is local and it usually affects the lower extremities, only rarely affecting other body areas. It is usually called pretibial myxedema due to its localization. The pathogenesis of pretibial myxedema remains not entirely known. Its pathogenesis has not been adequately investigated and clarified. It is observed in 0.05–4.3% of patients with Graves' disease. In patients with severe ophthalmopathy up to 13% of patients may develop myxedema [9, 10].

Myxedema may be asymmetric, brown with palpable limits and appears with various clinical presentations in the lower extremities. Myxedema may be diffuse, edematous and may be due to lymphatic press and occlusion and the presence of glycosaminoglycans. It may take the form of raised plaques in the presence of edema. It may take the form of nodular lesions. In very rare cases it may take the form of elephantiasis, nodular lesions with lymphedema.

Thyroid acropathy is a rare manifestation of Graves' disease and it is observed in 0.1–1% of patients with Graves' disease. Almost all patients with thyroid acropathy have thyroid ophthalmopathy and pretibial myxedema. The most common clinical manifestation of thyroid acropathy is plectrodactyly affecting hands and feet [11]. Fibrosis and periosteal bone formation in the digits, the metacarpal bones and metatarsal bones may be observed. It usually is not symptomatic and does not cause deformity. The pathogenesis of thyroid acropathy is not known and there appears to be no known effective treatment.

3. Pathophysiology

Graves' disease is an autoimmune disease. Antibodies against TSH receptors (TRAbs) are formed and stimulate the respective receptors, activate adenylate cyclase and increase the production of thyroid hormones, increase thyroid size and vascularization [12]. The etiology of Graves' disease is related to genetic factors and the effects of environmental and endogenous factors. Etiology is thought to be related to genetic susceptibility and the effect of environmental factors or endogenous factors [3] (**Figure 1**). Both T and B lymphocytes are involved in its pathogenesis [13, 14].

T lymphocytes are involved in the pathogenesis of Graves' disease [13]. In particular, Tregs appear to be lower in the circulation of Graves' disease patients [15, 16]. Alterations in Treg frequency or function are implicated in Graves' disease pathogenesis [17]. In particular, it appears that Tregs tend to transit to subsets with proinflammatory phenotypes, such as Th17 and Th1 lymphocytes in Graves' disease [18]. This transition of Treg cells to subsets of T lymphocytes with proinflammatory properties may contribute to the impaired anti-inflammatory properties of Tregs in Graves' disease. B lymphocytes are involved in the secretion of TRabs in Graves' disease [19, 20].

It appears that in the pathogenesis of Graves' disease contributes the loss of both central and peripheral immune tolerance. Tregs contribute to immune tolerance. In Graves' disease, Tregs appear to be reduced in both number and function and may contribute to impaired immune regulation and the development of autoimmunity in genetically susceptible patients.

TSH receptor antibodies, including those of the neutral type, may be involved in reactive oxygen species induction and the pathogenesis of autoimmune inflammatory

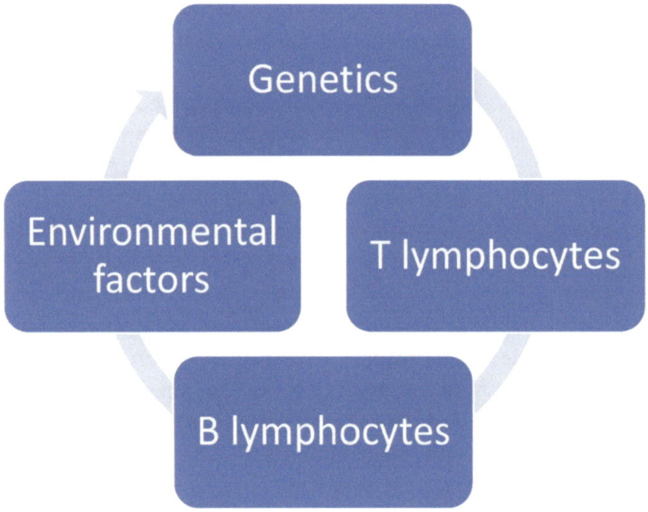

Figure 1.
Pathogenesis of Graves' disease.

reactions in Graves' disease [20]. Decreased interleukin-4 levels appear to be involved in the pathogenesis of Graves' disease [21]. Low serum interleukin-38 levels have been described in patients with Graves' disease [22]. TPO antibodies appear to display heterogeneity in the various forms of autoimmune thyroid disorders, including Graves' disease [23]. A possible interplay between estrogen and B-cell activating factor may exist and may be responsible for the higher incidence of Graves' disease in female patients [24].

4. Clinical presentation

Severity of symptoms and signs of hyperthyroidism is related to disease duration, the degree of the increase in thyroid hormone levels and patient age [13, 22–24].

One of the commonest findings of hyperthyroidism is weight loss despite normal food intake and normal appetite. Weight loss leads to loss of the deposited adipose tissue and loss of muscular mass. The increased metabolic rate which is the result of hyperthyroidism with increased energy production, leads to increased thermal energy production, increased body temperature, increased perspiration, heat intolerance and mildly increased body temperature. Patients exhibit generalized muscular weakness due to myopathy. Very rarely, periodic thyrotoxic paralysis may be observed which is characterized by episodes of muscular paralysis with hypokalemia and hyperthyroidism. Periodic thyrotoxic paralysis affects mainly patients of Chinese or Japanese origin [25–29].

Thyroid hormones affect the vascular system and the heart. They decrease vascular resistance *via* vasodilatory action on vascular smooth muscles *via* release of nitric oxide and various vasodilatory substances [30]. T_3 exerts its effects directly on the heart *via* various genetic effects acting on the production of various proteins of the muscular fibers, the calcium-dependent ATPase and various transfer mechanisms of the plasma membrane. T_3 acts additionally *via* non-genetic effects acting on sodium, potassium and calcium receptors. T_3 increases cardiac rhythm and cardiac contractility [31–33]. The most frequent symptom of hyperthyroidism is tachycardia. Tachycardia is observed in clinical examination in more than 90% of patients. Atrial fibrillation is observed in up to 20% of elderly patients as compared to 1.8% of young patients. Cardiac hypertrophy may be observed in patients on long-term hyperthyroidism who have not undergone proper treatment [34–37]. Arterial hypertension may be observed, with increased systolic and decreased diastolic pressure. Pulmonary hypertension may be observed in up to 47% of patients based on cardiac ultrasonography [38, 39]. Hyperthyroidism may be accompanied by increased demand on myocardial oxygenation and contraction of the coronary arteries and may lead to coronary ischemia and ischemic cardiac disease. Cardiac insufficiency may also be observed in elderly patients [40].

Hyperthyroidism may be accompanied by gastrointestinal manifestations such as increased gut motility which may sometimes lead to diarrhea [41]. Hyperthyroidism may also be accompanied by neuropsychiatric manifestations such as stress, anxiety and sentimental instability which may lead to frank psychosis in some rare cases [42]. Disorders of memory and concentration have also been observed. Hyperthyroidism may be accompanied by menstrual disorders in female patients and by gynecomastia or disorders of libido in male patients.

Thyroid ophthalmopathy is frequently observed in Graves' disease and is the most common extrathyroidal manifestation of Graves' disease. It is classified in six stages according to its severity from 0 which means lack of thyroid ophthalmopathy, to 6, which means ophthalmic nerve involvement. On clinical examination, goiter is usually observed in Graves' disease.

The impact of Graves' disease on bone metabolism has also been discussed extensively in the literature [43]. The relationship of Graves' disease with the development of lymphoma has also been discussed [44].

5. Laboratory evaluation

Diagnosis of hyperthyroidism is based on the measurement of thyroid hormones in the blood. Low TSH with high FT_4 is observed in 95% of patients with clinical signs of hyperthyroidism, while in some patients, FT_4 may be normal and FT_3 increased. Measurement of FT_3 and FT_4 is preferred over the measurement of T_3 and T_4, as a disorder may be observed in the conjugation of thyroid hormones to the proteins with which the hormones circulate bound, in particular thyroid binding globulin (TBG) and thyroid binding prealbumin (TBPA). Measurement of free thyroid hormones is absolutely necessary in viral hepatitis, pregnancy, and in patients taking estrogens. Measurement of free thyroid hormones is preferred as they are biologically active and reflect the metabolic situation. Thyroid antibodies and Trab should also be measured in Graves' disease.

6. Treatment

Treatment of Graves' disease is accomplished by the administration of antithyroid drugs, namely carbimazole, methimazole and propylthiouracil, administration of radioactive iodine and thyroidectomy. Antithyroid drugs block thyroid hormone synthesis. They are not characterized by severe adverse effects, however, treatment is chronic and eventually a block and replace regimen with antithyroid drugs and thyroxine may be needed. Radioiodine administration and thyroidectomy cause permanent hypothyroidism and lifelong thyroxine administration is necessary. However, nowadays, modern drugs based on the pathophysiology of the disease have entered the therapeutic landscape of Graves' disease.

Intravenous immunoglobulins and corticosteroids may reduce inflammation and ocular manifestations in patients with Graves' disease and Graves' ophthalmopathy. However, modern immune-modulating drugs have been shown to benefit patients with Graves' disease. Anti-TNF-a agents have been tested in Graves' disease. Etanercept, an anti-TNF-a agent, has been tested in Graves' ophthalmopathy [45, 46]. Rituximab, an anti-CD20 monoclonal antibody has also been tested in Graves' ophthalmopathy [47]. Tocilizumab, a monoclonal antibody against the IL-6 receptor, has also been tested and may be beneficial in Graves' ophthalmopathy [8, 48, 49]. Teprotumumab, a monoclonal antibody against IGF-1 receptor, is a promising therapy for Graves' disease. However, this treatment modality, although very promising, is characterized by cumbersome logistics [48, 50].

7. Future perspectives

The pathophysiology of Graves' disease although extensively investigated has not been fully elucidated. Further research is needed on it. Treatment of Graves' ophthalmopathy is under intense investigation and novel therapeutic agents are under evaluation.

8. Conclusion

In conclusion, Graves' disease is an autoimmune disease characterized by hyperthyroidism and extrathyroidal manifestations, namely, Graves' ophthalmopathy and acropathy. The disease is characterized by antibodies against the TSH receptor. Both T and B lymphocytes are involved in the pathogenesis of the disease. Antithyroid drugs, radioiodine administration and thyroidectomy are used in the treatment of the disease. Corticosteroids and modern biological agents, such as tocilizumab and teprotumumab, are now employed in the treatment of Graves' ophthalmopathy and hold promise in this area.

Conflict of interest

The authors declare no conflict of interest.

Author details

Ifigenia Kostoglou-Athanassiou[1*], Lambros Athanassiou[2] and Panagiotis Athanassiou[3]

1 Department of Endocrinology, Diabetes and Metabolism, Asclepeion Hospital, Voula, Athens, Greece

2 Department of Rheumatology, Asclepeion Hospital, Voula, Athens, Greece

3 Department of Rheumatology, St. Paul's Hospital, Thessaloniki, Greece

*Address all correspondence to: ikostoglouathanassiou@yahoo.gr

References

[1] Singer PA, Cooper DS, Levy EG, Ladenson PW, Braverman LE, Daniels G, et al. Treatment guidelines for patients with hyperthyroidism and hypothyroidism. Standards of Care Committee, American Thyroid Association. Journal of the American Medical Association. 1995;**273**(10):808-812

[2] Brownlie BE, Wells JE. The epidemiology of thyrotoxicosis in New Zealand: Incidence and geographical distribution in North Canterbury, 1983-1985. Clinical Endocrinology. 1990;**33**(2):249-259

[3] Lane LC, Cheetham TD, Perros P, Pearce SHS. New therapeutic horizons for Graves' hyperthyroidism. Endocrine Reviews. 2020;**41**(6):873-884

[4] Chiu HI, Wu SB, Tsai CC. The role of fibrogenesis and extracellular matrix proteins in the pathogenesis of Graves' ophthalmopathy. International Journal of Molecular Sciences. 2024;**25**(6):3288

[5] Velkeniers B, Salu P. Pathogenesis and treatment of the ophthalmopathy associated with Graves' disease. Bulletin de la Société Belge d'Ophtalmologie. 1992;**245**:9-14

[6] Prabhakar BS, Bahn RS, Smith TJ. Current perspective on the pathogenesis of Graves' disease and ophthalmopathy. Endocrine Reviews. 2003;**24**(6):802-835

[7] Bahn RS. Graves' ophthalmopathy. The New England Journal of Medicine. 2010;**362**(8):726-738

[8] Bartalena L, Tanda ML. Current concepts regarding Graves' orbitopathy. Journal of Internal Medicine. 2022;**292**(5):692-716

[9] Fatourechi V, Garrity JA, Bartley GB, Bergstralh EJ, Gorman CA. Orbital decompression in Graves' ophthalmopathy associated with pretibial myxedema. Journal of Endocrinological Investigation. 1993;**16**(6):433-437

[10] Lohiya S, Lohiya V, Stahl EJ. Pretibial myxedema without ophthalmopathy: An initial presentation of Graves' disease. The American Journal of the Medical Sciences. 2013;**346**(1):73-75

[11] Kelly DA, Turbin RE. Rapid response of thyroid eye disease, peripheral edema, and acropathy to teprotumumab infusion. American Journal of Ophthalmology Case Reports. 2024;**34**:102031

[12] Suzuki N, Inoue K, Yoshimura R, Kinoshita A, Suzuki A, Fukushita M, et al. The mediation role of thyrotropin receptor antibody in the relationship between age and severity of hyperthyroidism in Graves' disease. Thyroid. 2022;**32**(10):1243-1248

[13] Antonelli A, Fallahi P, Elia G, Ragusa F, Paparo SR, Ruffilli I, et al. Graves' disease: Clinical manifestations, immune pathogenesis (cytokines and chemokines) and therapy. Best Practice & Research. Clinical Endocrinology & Metabolism. 2020;**34**(1):101388

[14] Bartalena L. Diagnosis and management of Graves disease: A global overview. Nature Reviews. Endocrinology. 2013;**9**(12):724-734

[15] Liu Z, Ke SR, Shi ZX, Zhou M, Sun L, Sun QH, et al. Dynamic transition of Tregs to cytotoxic phenotype amid systemic inflammation in Graves' ophthalmopathy. JCI Insight. 2024;**9**(22):e181488

[16] Chen Z, Wang Y, Ding X, Zhang M, He M, Zhao Y, et al. The proportion of peripheral blood Tregs among the CD4+ T cells of autoimmune thyroid disease patients: A meta-analysis. Endocrine Journal. 2020;**67**(3):317-326

[17] Kustrimovic N, Gallo D, Piantanida E, Bartalena L, Lai A, Zerbinati N, et al. Regulatory T cells in the pathogenesis of Graves' disease. International Journal of Molecular Sciences. 2023;**24**(22):16432

[18] Fountoulakis S, Vartholomatos G, Kolaitis N, Frillingos S, Philippou G, Tsatsoulis A. HLA-DR expressing peripheral T regulatory cells in newly diagnosed patients with different forms of autoimmune thyroid disease. Thyroid. 2008;**18**(11):1195-1200

[19] Barros Silva AC, Damas II, Moma CA, Barreto IS, Zantut-Wittmann DE. Lower proportion of intra-thyroidal B lymphocytes CD20(+) associated to methimazole and lack of influence of iodide on lymphocyte subpopulations in Graves' disease. Molecular and Cellular Endocrinology. 2024;**592**:112331

[20] Kristensen B, Hegedüs L, Lundy SK, Brimnes MK, Smith TJ, Nielsen CH. Characterization of regulatory B cells in Graves' disease and Hashimoto's thyroiditis. PLoS ONE. 2015;**10**(5):e0127949

[21] Gong L, Huang G, Weng L, Xu J, Li Y, Cui W, et al. Decreased serum interleukin-41/Metrnl levels in patients with Graves' disease. Journal of Clinical Laboratory Analysis. 2022;**36**(10):e24676

[22] Ross DS, Burch HB, Cooper DS, Greenlee MC, Laurberg P, Maia AL, et al. 2016 American Thyroid Association guidelines for diagnosis and management of hyperthyroidism and other causes of thyrotoxicosis. Thyroid. 2016;**26**(10):1343-1421

[23] Bartalena L, Kahaly GJ, Baldeschi L, Dayan CM, Eckstein A, Marcocci C, et al. The 2021 European Group on Graves' orbitopathy (EUGOGO) clinical practice guidelines for the medical management of Graves' orbitopathy. European Journal of Endocrinology. 2021;**185**(4):G43-g67

[24] Hoang TD, Stocker DJ, Chou EL, Burch HB. 2022 update on clinical management of Graves disease and thyroid eye disease. Endocrinology and Metabolism Clinics of North America. 2022;**51**(2):287-304

[25] Siddamreddy S, Dandu VH. Thyrotoxic periodic paralysis. In: StatPearls. Treasure Island (FL): StatPearls Publishing LLC; 2025

[26] Lin SH. Thyrotoxic periodic paralysis. Mayo Clinic Proceedings. 2005;**80**(1):99-105

[27] Patel M, Ladak K. Thyrotoxic periodic paralysis: A case report and literature review. Clinical Medicine & Research. 2021;**19**(3):148-151

[28] Fialho D, Griggs RC, Matthews E. Periodic paralysis. Handbook of Clinical Neurology. 2018;**148**:505-520

[29] Iqbal QZ, Niazi M, Zia Z, Sattar SBA. A literature review on thyrotoxic periodic paralysis. Cureus. 2020;**12**(8):e10108

[30] Klein I, Danzi S. Thyroid disease and the heart. Circulation. 2007;**116**(15):1725-1735

[31] Athanasios T, Antonios B, Antonios L, Eustathios K, Maria G, Despina P. T3 and cardiac myocyte cell: A theoretical model. Recent Patents on Cardiovascular Drug Discovery. 2013;**8**(2):162-165

[32] Moolman JA. Thyroid hormone and the heart. Cardiovascular Journal of South Africa. 2002;**13**(4):159-163

[33] Witczak JK, Ubaysekara N, Ravindran R, Rice S, Yousef Z, Premawardhana LD. Significant cardiac disease complicating Graves' disease in previously healthy young adults. Endocrinology, Diabetes & Metabolism Case Reports. 2020;**2020**:19-0132

[34] Reddy V, Taha W, Kundumadam S, Khan M. Atrial fibrillation and hyperthyroidism: A literature review. Indian Heart Journal. 2017;**69**(4):545-550

[35] Higa S, Maesato A, Ishigaki S, Suenari K, Chen YJ, Chen SA. Diabetes and endocrine disorders (hyperthyroidism/hypothyroidism) as risk factors for atrial fibrillation. Cardiac Electrophysiology Clinics. 2021;**13**(1):63-75

[36] Kostopoulos G, Effraimidis G. Epidemiology, prognosis, and challenges in the management of hyperthyroidism-related atrial fibrillation. European Thyroid Journal. 2024;**13**(2):e230254

[37] Ellervik C, Roselli C, Christophersen IE, Alonso A, Pietzner M, Sitlani CM, et al. Assessment of the relationship between genetic determinants of thyroid function and atrial fibrillation: A Mendelian randomization study. JAMA Cardiology. 2019;**4**(2):144-152

[38] Vallabhajosula S, Radhi S, Cevik C, Alalawi R, Raj R, Nugent K. Hyperthyroidism and pulmonary hypertension: An important association. The American Journal of the Medical Sciences. 2011;**342**(6):507-512

[39] Itagaki T, Miura T, Kasai T, Ikeda U. Symptomatic and severe pulmonary hypertension due to hyperthyroidism. BML Case Reports. 2022;**15**(8):e251120

[40] Osuna PM, Udovcic M, Sharma MD. Hyperthyroidism and the heart. Methodist DeBakey Cardiovascular Journal. 2017;**13**(2):60-63

[41] Ebert EC. The thyroid and the gut. Journal of Clinical Gastroenterology. 2010;**44**(6):402-406

[42] Jurado-Flores M, Warda F, Mooradian A. Pathophysiology and clinical features of neuropsychiatric manifestations of thyroid disease. Journal of the Endocrine Society. 2022;**6**(2):bvab194

[43] Khamisi S, Udumyan R, Sjölin G, Calissendorff J, Filipsson Nyström H, Holmberg M, et al. Fracture incidence in Graves' disease: A population-based study. Thyroid. 2023;**33**(11):1349-1357

[44] Suzuki N, Watanabe N, Noh JY, Yoshimura R, Mikura K, Kinoshita A, et al. The relationship between primary thyroid lymphoma and various types of thyroid autoimmunity: A retrospective cohort study of 498 cases, including 9 cases with Graves' disease. Thyroid. 2022;**32**(5):552-559

[45] Elia G, Fallahi P, Ragusa F, Paparo SR, Mazzi V, Benvenga S, et al. Precision medicine in Graves' disease and ophthalmopathy. Frontiers in Pharmacology. 2021;**12**:754386

[46] Boskovic O, Medenica S, Radojevic N, Zarkovic M. Etanercept in the treatment of Graves' ophthalmopathy with primary hypothyroidism and rheumatoid arthritis. Central European Journal of Immunology. 2019;**44**(4):463-465

[47] Supronik J, Szelachowska M, Kretowski A, Siewko K. Rituximab in the

treatment of Graves' orbitopathy: Latest updates and perspectives. Endocrine Connections. 2022;**11**(12):e220303

[48] Taylor PN, Zhang L, Lee RWJ, Muller I, Ezra DG, Dayan CM, et al. New insights into the pathogenesis and nonsurgical management of Graves orbitopathy. Nature Reviews. Endocrinology. 2020;**16**(2):104-116

[49] Duarte AF, Xavier NF, Sales Sanz M, Cruz AAV. Efficiency and safety of tocilizumab for the treatment of thyroid eye disease: A systematic review. Ophthalmic Plastic & Reconstructive Surgery. 2024;**40**(4):367-373

[50] Douglas RS, Couch S, Wester ST, Fowler BT, Liu CY, Subramanian PS, et al. Efficacy and safety of teprotumumab in patients with thyroid eye disease of long duration and low disease activity. The Journal of Clinical Endocrinology and Metabolism. 2023;**109**(1):25-35

Chapter 6

Radioiodine Treatment for Hyperthyroid Graves' Disease

Yongji Jiang and Chao Ma

Abstract

Hyperthyroidism is an endocrine disease caused by the inappropriate and continuous synthesis and secretion of excessive thyroid hormones by the thyroid gland, and the most common cause is Graves' disease (GD). The diagnosis of GD is mainly based on clinical symptoms, signs and thyroid function. Antithyroid drugs (ATD), radioiodine (RAI) and surgery are all effective treatments for GD. In recent decades, the preferred treatment methods for GD in various countries have also changed, and more and more people choose ATD as their first choice of treatment. Hypothyroidism, occurrence and progression of Graves' orbitopathy (GO), and other side effects after RAI treatment has limited its application to a certain extent. However, RAI treatment is still a safe, cost-effective and long-lasting treatment option for GD, and its usage, benefits and risks are gradually being understood.

Keywords: Graves' disease, hyperthyroidism, radioiodine, RAI treatment, efficacy

1. Introduction

Hyperthyroidism is an endocrine disease caused by excessive production and secretion of thyroid hormone by the thyroid gland. The most common causes are Graves' disease and toxic nodular goiter, of which GD accounts for approximately 70–80% [1, 2]. GD is characterized by suppressed serum thyroid stimulating hormone (TSH) concentrations, accompanied by elevated free thyroxine (FT_4) and free triiodothyronine (FT_3) concentrations. Treatment options for GD have remained essentially unchanged for the past 80 years. Once GD is diagnosed, patients and physicians must choose one of three effective and relatively safe initial treatment options: RAI, ATD, or thyroidectomy treatment. Despite improvements in administration and safety, current treatment approaches have significant limitations, particularly high relapse rates after discontinuation of ATD and hypothyroidism after RAI or surgery treatment.

In recent decades, the preferred treatment for GD has also changed in various countries, with ATD increasingly being the first choice for GD treatment rather than RAI and surgery [3]. Current guidelines recommend a course of ATD for 12–18 months, firstly in GD patients [4, 5]. Clinicians in Europe and the Asia Pacific generally prefer ATD as first-line therapy [6, 7]. The most significant decline in the use of RAI for hyperthyroidism occurred in the United States over the past two decades, with the preferred treatment changing to ATD rather than RAI, from 69% in 1990 to 59.7% in 2012 [7, 8]. Other recent surveys have reported only 7–35% of patients are willing to choose RAI treatment for hyperthyroidism [3, 9]. The main reasons for this change include (1) a desire to avoid hypothyroidism, (2) a desire to achieve a remission, (3) to avoid exposure to RAI and (4) to avoid worsening GO related to RAI therapy, the most important of which is the desire to avoid hypothyroidism [3]. Approximately 50–85% of GD patients will develop hypothyroidism after RAI treatment and will develop at a rate of 2–5% per year [10, 11]. Hypothyroidism that occurs within 1 year after treatment is related to the RAI dose. The higher the dose, the higher the one-time remission rate and the higher the incidence of early hypothyroidism, and this is both the advantage and disadvantage of RAI treatment. An appropriate RAI dose is to control hyperthyroidism as much as possible while avoiding radiation risks. RAI treatment may cause worsening of existing GO or develop new GO, which is also a problem that needs to be considered. In the past decade, many clinical studies and meta-analyses have reported an increasing trend in the incidence and mortality of tumors after RAI treatment for hyperthyroidism, and the risk of cardio-cerebrovascular diseases is also gradually increasing [12, 13]. However, many scholars disagree with these views and believe that there is no clear relationship between RAI treatment in hyperthyroidism and these side effects. This article discusses this in detail under the title "Side effects," but it does not mean that the side effects of RAI treatment for GD are completely clear. Overall, RAI treatment is still a safe, cost-effective and long-lasting treatment.

2. RAI treatment principle

Iodine is an essential raw material for the synthesis of thyroid hormones, and it is taken up by thyroid follicular cells via the sodium-iodine-symporter (NIS), then is incorporated into thyroglobulin and stored in the thyroid follicles. GD patients are usually accompanied by high thyroid radioactive iodine uptake (RAIU). So, the thyroid gland can absorb most of the administered RAI.

Iodine-131 (^{131}I) is one kind of RAI, and it is widely used for GD treatment. The decay process of ^{131}I can release both β and γ rays, and the β ray is used for radiotherapy. Due to its high mean energy (190 keV), ^{131}I has a mean biological tissue penetration of 0.8 mm (0.6–2 mm) [14]. About 90% of ^{131}I energy is absorbed within 0.8 mm by thyroid cells [15]. β rays have a strong penetration ability and damage cells directly, which can cause degeneration and necrosis of thyroid follicular cells and reduce the synthesis and secretion of thyroid hormones. The half-life of ^{131}I is about 8.0 days, but the effective half-life in the thyroid gland ranges from 1.9 to 7.9 days in different studies, and the sustained effect of a single therapeutic dose of ^{131}I on the thyroid gland can reach 30–60 days [14, 16, 17]. Subsequently, the volume of the thyroid gland is reduced, and the function is weakened; the purpose of GD treatment is achieved.

3. Indications and contraindications for RAI treatment

With a deeper knowledge of thyroid disease, the treatment concept is constantly updated. The clinical practice of RAI treatment for GD has changed substantially in recent years. Patient conditions (thyroid volume size, severity of the disease, disease duration, with or without complications, psychiatric and psychological conditions, pregnancy or lactation status, birth plan), treatment costs and available medical resources should all be taken into account when choosing among treatments. Physicians need to communicate adequately with patients, weigh the pros and cons and make the most appropriate clinical treatment decision. There are no absolute indications for RAI treatment for GD. Indications and contraindications for GD RAI treatment are as follows [4, 5, 10, 14].

3.1 Indications

a. Adverse drug reactions associated with ATD

b. Poor ATD efficacy or multiple recurrences after ATD treatment

c. At high surgical risk or with contraindications to surgery

d. History of neck irradiation or neck surgery

e. Long disease duration of GD

f. Elderly patients, especially combined with cardiovascular disease

g. Combined with liver function damage, leukopenia or thrombocytopenia, skeletal muscle periodic hypokalemic paralysis, atrial fibrillation, right heart failure pulmonary hypertension, or congestive heart failure

h. Women planning a pregnancy in the future (in more than 6 months following RAI treatment, provided thyroid hormone levels are normal)

3.2 Contraindications

a. Pregnancy or lactation (absolute contraindications)

b. Combined with suspected or definite thyroid cancer

c. Individuals unable to adhere to radiation safety guidelines

d. Women planning a pregnancy within 4–6 months

e. Moderate-to-severe or sight-threatening active GO

4. Indications of ATD before and after RAI treatment

Given that hyperthyroidism symptoms may worsen in the short term after RAI treatment, ATD pretreatment before RAI treatment should be considered. Especially for severe illness, elderly, combined with significantly elevated serum FT_4 (greater than two to three times the normal upper limit value), and complications risk increased with worsening of hyperthyroidism. The patient's condition should be stabilized as much as possible before RAI treatment. There is no standard consensus on the optimal time of ATD discontinuation before RAI treatment. Methimazole (MMI) is the first choice for treatment, and it should be discontinued 2–7 days before RAI treatment, while propylthiouracil should be discontinued 1–2 weeks [5, 14, 18]. For young and middle-aged GD patients with mild clinical symptoms, RAI treatment can be performed directly without ATD, even if the FT_4 level is high.

For GD patients with severe illness or combined with complications or comorbidities, ATD (methimazole is preferred) should be continued to be administered to control symptoms 3–7 days after RAI treatment. In the following 4–6 weeks, when FT_4 tends to be normal, the ATD should be gradually reduced and discontinued [5].

A meta-analysis reported that if ATD is given before, with, or after RAI treatment, the treatment failures increase [Relative risk (RR) 1.28, 95% CI 1.07–1.52] and the risk of hypothyroidism reduces [RR 0.68, 95% CI 0.53–0.87], especially if ATD are given with or after RAI treatment [19]. The probable explanation may be pretreatment with ATD potentially decreases the uptake of RAI and this could be overridden by increasing the RAI dose. It is also reported that 4 days of MMI discontinuation is enough and can eliminate any effect of MMI on therapy success [20]. 24–48 hours of MMI discontinuation before RAI uptake measurement (38–72 hours) may also be effective as longer MMI discontinuation [18].

5. Indications of β-adrenergic receptor blockade before and after RAI treatment

β-Adrenergic receptor blockade can control heart rate and systolic blood pressure, improve muscle weakness and tremor and improve the severity of irritability, emotional instability and exercise intolerance [21], which include non-selective blockade (representative drugs: propranolol and nadolol) and selective β1 receptor blockade (representative drugs: metoprolol, atenolol, bisoprolol, etc.) [22].

a. Propranolol has the most applied experience, and it is recommended 10–40 mg, three to four times per day. It can prevent FT_4 to FT_3 conversion at high doses (40 mg, four times per day).

b. Nadolol is recommended 40–160 mg, one time per day; it has the least experience to date and may prevent FT_4 to FT_3 conversion at high doses.

c. Atenolol is recommended 25–100 mg, one to two times per day, and it should be avoided during pregnancy.

d. Metoprolol is recommended 25–50 mg, two to three times per day.

If there are no medication contraindications, GD patients can use β-adrenergic receptor blockade before RAI treatment, especially elderly patients, or a resting heart rate > 90 beats/min, or combined with cardiovascular and other systemic diseases [14]. Notably, propranolol should not be used in patients with bronchial asthma.

In the early stage (1–2 weeks) after RAI treatment for GD, thyroid hormone stored in the follicles is released into the blood due to radiation thyroiditis, which can aggravate the symptoms of hypermetabolism. In the absence of contraindications, β-adrenergic receptor blockade can be used for all GD patients, especially elderly patients and GD patients with a resting heart rate > 90 beats/min or combined with cardiovascular diseases. For a period of time after RAI treatment, the use of β-adrenergic receptor blockade can effectively relieve symptoms and reduce the occurrence of complications [21, 23]. With the relief of symptoms, β-adrenergic receptor blockade can be reduced and discontinued.

6. Dose determination for RAI treatment

6.1 Determination of thyroid volume

Determination of RAI dose usually requires assessment of thyroid volume and weight. The three-dimensional method is often used to measure the volume of the thyroid gland by ultrasound. L represents the length of one lobe of the thyroid gland, W represents the width, and T represents the thickness (all in centimeters). The volume of one lobe is calculated using the following formula: $V = \pi/6 \cdot L \cdot W \cdot T$. The sum of the volumes of two lobes is total volume of thyroid gland, and the weight of the thyroid gland (g) is calculated, taking 1.0 as specific gravity [24].

The formula for calculating the thyroid volume by thyroid radionuclide imaging is V = average height of two lobes (cm) × frontal projection area of two lobes (cm^2) × K (K is a constant, ranging from 0.23 to 0.32, and varies with different imaging conditions). Thyroid radionuclide imaging is susceptible to many factors, such as thyroid size, gland thickness and the ratio of gland to background radioactivity [25]. Thyroid palpation can assist in determining the volume and make up for the inadequacy of thyroid radionuclide imaging in assessing thyroid weight. The palpation is of great value in assessing thyroid texture and the presence of nodules and adjusting the RAI treatment dose.

6.2 Determination of RAI dose

There are two methods for determining the RAI dose for GD treatment: the calculated dose method and the fixed dose method.

1. Calculated dose approach. The dose is calculated based on the thyroid weight and RAIU. The dose per gram of thyroid tissue usually ranges from 1.85 to 7.40 MBq (50–200 μCi). Oral RAI activity (MBq or μCi) = [planned dose (MBq or μCi/g) × thyroid weight (g)]/[maximum RAIU or 24 h RAIU (%)]. This formula is based on the assumption that the effective half-life of RAI in the thyroid is 5 days. If the effective half-life varies greatly, the RAI dose should also be adjusted accordingly.

2. Fixed dose approach. A fixed dose is given at one time based on the volume and weight of the thyroid gland. For example, for patients with thyroid grade-I enlargement, 185 MBq RAI can be given; for grade-II enlargement, 370 MBq; for grade-III enlargement, 555–1110 MBq [14]. The American Thyroid Association (ATA) recommends fixed RAI activities of 370–555 MBq for GD, and the Royal College of Physicians UK guidelines 2007 recommends 400–600 MBq for uncomplicated GD patients [5, 26]. The 2018 European Thyroid Association guideline comments that providing a fixed activities RAI is still fully acceptable because "no dose calculation can secure long-term euthyroidism" [4]. This method is simple and has a high one-time remission rate.

The advantage of the calculated dose approach is that it can reduce the dose of RAI, especially for GD patients with smaller thyroid glands. The fixed dose approach is easy to operate and master. It is currently believed that the overall efficacy of calculated dose method and fixed dose method are generally equivalent in determining the dose of RAI for GD patients [27–29]. It has also been reported that the fixed-dose regimen showed a significant advantage compared with the calculated dose and has a higher success rate and a lower incidence of persistent hyperthyroidism [30].

6.3 RAI dose adjustment

Iodine-rich foods and seaweed health products should be avoided 1–2 weeks before RAI treatment. Iodine-containing contrast agents and drugs (amiodarone, etc.) should also be avoided. Regardless of which dose method is used, the following factors can be taken into consideration to adjust the dose before RAI treatment. For GD patients with repeated relapses and long disease duration, the goal of RAI is to achieve hypothyroidism.

6.3.1 Increase the RAI dose

a. Larger thyroid volume and harder texture

b. Older age, longer disease course, or a history of long-term ATD use

c. Shorter effective half-life

d. Poor or ineffective after the first RAI treatment

e. Combined with cardiovascular disease, abnormal liver function, or leukopenia

6.3.2 Reduce the RAI dose

a. Shorter disease course, smaller thyroid volume and softer texture

b. No related treatment or relapse after surgery

c. Longer effective half-life

d. Significant efficacy after RAI treatment without complete remission

6.4 Other specific conditions

1. Upon combined with severe abnormalities in the hematopoietic system, multidisciplinary diagnosis and treatment should be carried out. When the condition tends to be stable, sufficient RAI should be performed to achieve hypothyroidism. RAI is mainly taken up by the hyperfunctioning thyroid tissue, and the irradiation dose to the bone marrow is small, which will not cause a further decrease in white blood cells and platelets.

2. For GD with atrial fibrillation, RAI treatment should be performed as soon as possible, with hypothyroidism as the treatment goal. Before treatment, a comprehensive assessment of cardiac function should be conducted. Timely cooperation with the cardiology department and correct complications such as atrial fibrillation and heart failure are necessary. As thyroid function returns to normal, paroxysmal atrial fibrillation may disappear. For patients with persistent atrial

fibrillation, sinus rhythm may restore in some cases. Regularly follow-up and correct hypothyroidism timely, and the impact on the heart will be reduced [31].

3. GD combined with abnormal liver function is related to many factors and can be divided into hyperthyroidism-induced liver injury, hyperthyroidism combined with other diseases that cause abnormal liver function, and ATD-related liver injury. The treatment principle is to target the cause and provide liver protection therapy. According to the degree and cause of liver damage, ATD should be decided whether to continue for those with severe liver damage, liver protection therapy should be carried out [32, 33]. When combined with severe hyperbilirubinemia or cholestatic hepatitis, the artificial liver support system can effectively improve the patient's clinical prognosis [34]. When liver function tends to be stable, sufficient RAI should be used as soon as possible, and the aim is to achieve hypothyroidism. RAI is mainly absorbed by thyroid tissue, and the liver absorbs rare RAI, in addition, and is insensitive to radiation, so RAI treatment will not further aggravate liver damage. Most patients with GD combined with liver damage can gradually return to normal liver function after their thyroid function is effectively controlled.

4. Currently, the single RAI treatment dose >1110 MBq (30 mCi) is not recommended. For patients with giant thyroid glands, if the calculated or estimated dose is >30 mCi, RAI needs to be divided into 2 or more doses, but this may also make the efficacy worse. Some scholars have shared their experience in treating hyperthyroidism with high single-dose RAI (1850–3700 MBq, 50–100 mCi) in some conferences and practices and have achieved good treatment results; after treatment, the patients are in good health.

7. The therapeutic effects of RAI treatment

7.1 Therapeutic effects

There is no absolutely ideal RAI dose for GD treatment that can correct hyperthyroidism without causing hypothyroidism. The criteria for the efficacy of RAI treatment for GD include the following [14]:

a. Complete remission or clinical recovery: the symptoms and signs of hyperthyroidism completely disappear, and the serum FT_4 level returns to normal after a follow-up of more than half a year.

b. Hypothyroidism: the related symptoms and signs appear, the serum FT_4 level is lower than normal, and the TSH is higher than normal.

c. Partial remission: the symptoms of hyperthyroidism are alleviated, the related signs partially disappear and the serum FT_4 level decreases but does not return to normal.

d. Ineffectiveness: the related symptoms and signs do not improve or even worsen, and the serum FT_4 level does not change significantly.

e. Relapse: the reappearance of hyperthyroidism symptoms and signs and the re-increase of serum FT_4 level after complete remission of RAI treatment.

GD patients are considered cured if persistent hypothyroidism or euthyroidism appears after RAI treatment. The dose of RAI used in GD varies between centers, with cure rates (persistent hypothyroidism and euthyroidism) ranging from 70% to 95% [22, 28, 35, 36]. The success of RAI treatment for GD depends largely on the dose administered. In most patients, thyroid function returns to normal within 4–8 weeks after RAI treatment, and the clinical symptoms improve. 50–90% of patients achieve euthyroidism within 3–12 months of RAI treatment [11]. T_4 and T_3 levels may increase temporarily in the first few weeks after RAI treatment, but eventually, 50–85% or more GD patients will develop hypothyroidism [37, 38], more commonly when a high RAI dose is administered. The incidence of hypothyroidism is 5–50% in the first year after RAI treatment. Hypothyroidism may occur from 4 weeks on, with 40% of patients developing hypothyroidism by 8 weeks and more than 80% by 16 weeks [39]. The incidence of hypothyroidism is 2–5% per year thereafter and is generally unrelated to RAI dose [11, 40]. Approximately 10–25% of patients will not alleviate after RAI treatment, depending on the underlying cause [11, 38]. The relapse rate of GD after RAI treatment is approximately 1–4% [41].

7.2 Influencing factors of therapeutic effects

Many factors can affect the therapeutic effects of RAI. Multiple studies reported that patients who are young or have lower thyroid weight, lower free thyroxine and TRAb levels, higher TPOAb levels, shorter disease duration and ATD administered duration, higher 24 h RAUI, higher RAI absorbed dose, and no smoking are more likely to be cured by RAI [42–51]. The current controversy is the high incidence of hypothyroidism after RAI treatment. There is also controversy regarding the use of low-dose or high-dose RAI for GD. The fixed-dose regimen uses a larger RAI dose than the calculated dose approach, so GD patients are more likely to be cured, but this is also accompanied by a higher likelihood of hypothyroidism and increased radiation exposure [28–30, 52]. Although the higher RAI doses are associated with high success rate, unnecessary radiation dose absorption must be strictly controlled according to the "as low as reasonably achievable" (ALARA) principle [53]. The American Thyroid Association recommends an average RAI dose of 370–555 MBq to achieve hypothyroidism in GD patients [5].

7.3 Treatment of different outcomes after RAI treatment

7.3.1 Hypothyroidism

Fatigue, lethargy, weight gain, chills, constipation and menstrual abnormalities in females after RAI treatment indicate the possibility of hypothyroidism and the need to recheck in time. When FT_4 is lower than the normal range and TSH is still suppressed, hypothyroidism should be considered. TSH level may not rise immediately as hypothyroidism develops and therefore should not be used initially to determine the need for levothyroxine. Hypothyroidism in some patients is temporary, and thyroid function can return to normal afterward. Upon hypothyroidism, levothyroxine is preferred for replacement therapy and drug dosage should be adjusted according to FT_4 levels. The timing of replacement therapy depends on thyroid function, clinical symptoms and physical examination. The dosage should be adjusted under the guidance of the physician to maintain normal FT_4 levels, and regular follow-up should be maintained during the replacement therapy [14].

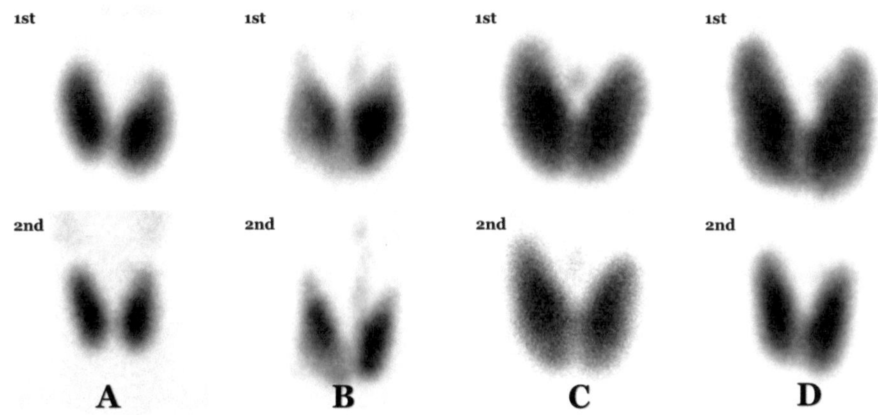

Figure 1.
Four GD patients with large goiter received twice RAI treatments, respectively, who evolved to hypothyroidism and then treated with levothyroxine. (A) A 44-year-old female received 8 and 6 mCi RAI, respectively. (B) A 39-year-old male received 9 and 8 mCi RAI, respectively. (C) A 28-year-old female received 18 and 23 mCi RAI, respectively. (D) A 30-year-old female received 15 and 10 mCi RAI, respectively.

7.3.2 Partial remission, ineffectiveness and relapse

For those whose symptoms and signs do not relieve or have been confirmed ineffective after 3 months follow-up, RAI can be used again. Once used again, the RAI dose can be appropriately increased for patients who are ineffective to previous treatment or with complications. A small number of GD patients with larger and harder thyroid glands require multiple RAI treatments to achieve complete remission (**Figure 1**). A study reported that for patients with post-RAI relapse of hyperthyroidism, long-term methimazole treatment was superior to RAI because of faster achievement of euthyroidism and more sustained control of hyperthyroidism during 60 months of follow-up [54]. For GD patients who are ineffective at RAI treatment or relapse after multiple RAI treatments, surgical treatment should be recommended. GD patients with normal FT_4 levels and persistently suppressed TSH need to be closely monitored to prevent conversion to clinical GD.

8. Graves' orbitopathy (GO)

Graves' orbitopathy, also called thyroid-associated ophthalmopathy (TAO) or thyroid eye disease (TED), is an organ-specific autoimmune disease closely related to thyroid disease. It ranks first in the incidence of adult orbital diseases and is also the most common extrathyroidal manifestation of GD, accounting for 25–40% of GD [55]. About 40% of GO patients develop eye disease after hyperthyroidism, about 40% develop eye disease and hyperthyroidism at the same time, and about 20% develop eye disease before hyperthyroidism [56]. The staging and grading of GO, as well as RAI-related treatment methods and developments, will be discussed below.

8.1 Staging and grading of GO

GO is an organ-specific autoimmune inflammatory reaction with a long course, which is divided into active and inactive stages. Patients may gradually enter the inactive stage after an active stage of 18–24 months [55]. The clinical activity score (CAS) is used to stage the disease activity of patients with newly diagnosed GO [22]. It includes seven items: spontaneous retrobulbar pain, pain on attempted upward or downward gaze, redness of eyelids, redness of conjunctiva, swelling of caruncle or plica, swelling of eyelids and swelling of conjunctiva (chemosis), each with 1 point. CAS ≥3 points is active GO and CAS <3 points are inactive GO. Staging assessment can combine the orbital MRI examination results and CAS. Staging GO activity can provide a basis for formulating treatment plans and evaluating prognosis.

The GO severity grading methods currently used in clinical practice mainly use the European Group on Graves' Orbitopathy (EUGOGO) grading, which can be used as a reference for clinical treatment plans. In 2016, EUGOGO proposed a grading standard for GO severity, which is mainly based on clinical symptoms, including eyelid retraction, proptosis, diplopia, optic nerve compression and corneal exposure lesions and is divided into three levels: mild, moderate-to-severe and sight threatening [22].

8.2 Management of GO

Thyroid dysfunction (including hyperthyroidism and hypothyroidism) affects the course of GO, therefore, rapid restoration and stable maintenance of euthyroidism is a priority. It is necessary to control risk factors throughout the process, maintain thyroid function stability and perform symptomatic supportive eye treatment at the same time.

Several studies have shown a significant association between RAI treatment and the development or progression of GO and the risk raging 10–39% [57–62]. Of course, some GD patients have improved hyperthyroidism and GO after RAI treatment. The progression of GO after RAI treatment has been attributed to post-treatment hypothyroidism and increased serum thyroid TRAb levels [63]. The point to note is the development or progression of GO is unrelated to RAI doses [59, 64]. GD patients combined GO can still select RAI treatment, specific treatment should be based on the patient's specific circumstances (**Table 1**) [4, 65–67].

For extremely severe GO patients who are sight-threatening, eye disease treatment should be given priority. If high-dose glucocorticoid shock therapy is ineffective for them, ophthalmic surgery should be performed as soon as possible. Numerous studies have shown that persistent, untreated hypothyroidism after treatment for hyperthyroidism has an adverse effect on the development of GO. One early study reported that GO was more severe in patients with hypothyroidism or hyperthyroidism than euthyroidism [68]. GO patients should restore their thyroid function as soon as possible, maintain stability and try to avoid hypothyroidism. Whether it is primary hypothyroidism, hypothyroidism after RAI treatment or thyroidectomy, levothyroxine should be given to correct it in time [65]. In addition to these, the related risk factors should also be controlled. Smoking can increase the incidence and severity of GO, and daily smoking amount is significantly related to the incidence of GO diplopia and proptosis symptoms [69]. Therefore, all GO patients, including active and passive smoking, should quit smoking and GD patients without GO should also quit smoking. RAI combined with ^{99}Tc-methylenediphosphonate (^{99}Tc-MDP) injection or selenium therapy may improve the remission rate of GO or prevent further aggravation of GO [70, 71]. The author is also currently conducting a clinical study to investigate whether ^{99}Tc-MDP can improve the remission rate of GD patients with mild-to-moderate GO and whether it can prevent the worsening of GO (Registration number: ChiCTR2200066740).

GD types	RAI treatment	Prevention or treatment measures for GO
GD (no GO)		
Low-risk	Yes	Glucocorticoids are not recommended
High-risk	Yes	A low dose of glucocorticoids can be used indeed: 0.1–0.2 mg/kg/d, gradually reduced and discontinued after 6 weeks
GD + GO		
Inactive GO (low-risk)	Yes	A low-dose of glucocorticoids: 0.1–0.2 mg/kg/d, gradually reduced and discontinued after 6 weeks; or not use glucocorticoids
Inactive GO (high-risk)	Yes	Glucocorticoids: 0.3–0.5 mg/kg/d, gradually reduced and discontinued after 3 months
Active GO (mild)	Yes	Glucocorticoids: 0.3–0.5 mg/kg/d, gradually reduced and discontinued after 3 months
Active GO (moderate-to-severe, sight threatening)	No	—
High-risk factors: smoking, severe hyperthyroidism, unstable thyroid function, high TRAb level and new GO; Low-risk factors: no smoking, long-term stable GO, low TRAb level		

Table 1.
RAI selection for different types of GD and prevention or treatment measures for GO.

9. Side effects

There will be some short- and long-term side effects after RAI treatment for GD. These are issues that patients may be anxious about, and physicians should also take those into consideration and inform patients and know how to deal with treatment-related adverse reactions and complications. GO has been mentioned before, and it will not be interpreted repeatedly here. Some potential side effects are described below, some of which are still controversial at this stage.

9.1 Short-time side effects and management

Most GD patients have no obvious clinical symptoms after RAI treatment. Some patients may develop fatigue, poor appetite, nausea, skin itching, thyroid swelling and other symptoms in the short term after RAI treatment, close observation and symptomatic management are suggested. A few patients may develop a close observation neck pain due to radiation thyroiditis, which may last for several weeks. Nonsteroidal anti-inflammatory drugs and glucocorticoids can be used to relieve regional pain. Though RAI treatment generally does not affect blood counts, some patients may develop a close observation of temporary leukopenia and drugs to increase leukocytes can be given if necessary.

9.2 Secondary malignancy

It has long been a common concern of radiation safety issues, and it limits the RAI application to a certain extent. It is generally accepted that the dose of RAI commonly used in GD produces a low radiation dose to patients and will not cause long-term radiation harm to patients. Whether RAI treatment for hyperthyroidism causes an increase in tumor incidence and tumor-specific mortality in patients with hyperthyroidism has been a constant concern for many years. Thyrotoxicosis Therapy Follow-up Study (TTFUS) reported the relationship between RAI treatment of hyperthyroidism and the risk of tumor occurrence and mortality in patients in 1968, 1974 and 1998, respectively [72–74]. The results showed that after RAI treatment for hyperthyroidism, the incidence of leukemia, the incidence of thyroid cancer and the overall cancer mortality rate did not increase significantly, indicating that RAI is a safe therapy option. A similar view that RAI is safe for patients with respect to carcinogenesis is reflected in recent society guidelines from both the ATA (2016) and the National Institute for Health and Care Excellence (United Kingdom, 2019) [5, 75]. In long-term follow-up, no association was found between RAI treatment for hyperthyroidism and risk for incident cancer [76–78].

In 2019, a new study of the cooperative TTFUS (CTTFUS) cohort sparked a heated debate about the safety of RAI treatment for hyperthyroidism. The study reanalyzed and expanded the CTTFUS cohort and found that higher estimated organ-absorbed doses of RAI were moderately positively associated with the risk of death from solid cancers, including breast cancer [12]. This conclusion has sparked a considerable critical response in nuclear medicine journals. Most prominently, nearly all questioned this dosimetric model and suggested it was not validated sufficiently to accept the dose-response results at face value. A linear dose-response association between RAI treatment and solid cancer mortality was also observed and some other previous studies found increased incidence or mortality from cancers of the kidney, breast, thyroid, non-Hodgkin's lymphoma, pulmonary, etc. [74, 76, 79–82].

Due to the lack of large randomized clinical trials on this topic, information on long-term associations of RAI treatment for GD with cancer and other outcomes has relied on results from observational studies. Results from the few previous large observational studies on this topic were discrepant and controversial. Overall, RAI is a safe and effective treatment for hyperthyroidism. Future studies should based on the foundation laid by previous studies and continually improve methods to make the study findings as clear and meaningful as possible.

9.3 Cerebrovascular and cardiovascular diseases

RAI treatment for benign thyroid disease exposes the carotid arteries to 4–50 Gy and may increase the risk of atherosclerosis. An increased risk of cerebrovascular events [hazard ratio (HR) 1.18, 95% CI 1.09–1.29] has been reported after RAI treatment for hyperthyroidism [13]. Nevertheless, another related study reported that patients with benign thyroid disease treated with RAI showed no early changes in carotid intima-media thickness (CIMT, progression of atherosclerosis can be examined by measuring CIMT) and indicated that RAI radiation has little or no effect on atherosclerosis in the carotid arteries [83].

Compared with surgery, RAI treatment for GD was associated with an increased risk of all-cause death [HR 0.82, 95% CI 0.71–0.96] during long-term follow-up. The difference in cardiovascular mortality between the two groups was the major cause. Men, in particular, appear to be at great risk [HR 0.46, 95% CI 0.31–0.68] when receiving RAI treatment for hyperthyroidism [84]. However, there were also cohort studies showed a significant reduction in overall risk of major adverse cardiovascular events in the surgery and RAI groups compared with the ATD group [85, 86].

The pathophysiology behind these increased cardio-cerebrovascular risks remains controversial, particularly whether these increased risks are related to thyroid disease itself or RAI treatment side effects, and it is worthy of continued study by researchers.

9.4 Reproductive and genetic security issues

The ovaries and testicles have low or no RAI uptake and RAI is excreted quickly in GD patients. RAI treatment will not damage the function of the testicles and ovaries, and patient's reproductive capacity will not be affected [87, 88]. The proportion of congenital malformations has not increased in the offspring of children and adolescent GD patients who received RAI treatment. The theoretical risk of genetic damage caused by RAI treatment is only 0.005%, while the spontaneous risk is 0.8% [89]. Checking thyroid function regularly, receiving antenatal care and maintaining good health during pregnancy, GD patients of childbearing age can deliver normally, and the newborns are as healthy as the general population [90, 91]. However, a large cohort study found that for women treated for GD or toxic multi- or uninodular goiter by RAI or surgery, the children born by them may have a lower birth weight, shorter birth length and average head circumference [92]. Considering the possible impact of abnormal thyroid function or radiation risk on pregnancy, GD patients, both genders, should consider pregnancy at least 6 months later after RAI treatment, when the thyroid hormone levels are normal.

9.5 Public radiation safety issue

Although GD patients receiving RAI treatment may cause a small amount of γ radiation to nearby people, and their excretions may also cause trace radiation contamination to the surrounding environment, the radiation is limited and will not cause radiation hazards to the surrounding people and the environment. The following radiation safety precautions should be followed when RAI is used for GD treatment: (1) After RAI treatment, it is advisable to drink more water and urinate more frequently. When defecating, the number of flushing times should be increased to avoid contamination of the feces with urine. (2) In order to ensure that the radiation dose to the public does not exceed 1 mSv, according to the relevant recommendations of the International Atomic Energy Agency publications, GD patients should avoid contact with colleagues, family members and children for a period of time after RAI treatment, based on the dose of RAI [93]. The above contents should be informed in detail by physicians to patients before treatment, and it is recommended to provide patients with written instruction materials.

10. Long-term follow-up after RAI treatment

After oral administration of RAI, the effect generally gradually occurs after 2–4 weeks, clinical symptoms are relieved, the thyroid volume is reduced and then the symptoms gradually disappear. FT_4 of most patients tends to be normal 8–12 weeks after RAI treatment. The remission rate of RAI treatment for GD is high, but those with too large and hard thyroid, or accompanied by nodules require multiple treatments to be cured. Follow-up after RAI treatment is an important part of GD patients. Patients with mild or moderate GD and no serious complications can be followed up 4–8 weeks after treatment to preliminarily evaluate the efficacy. For those with infiltrative exophthalmos, it is recommended to test FT_4 testing as soon as possible 4 weeks after RAI treatment, to avoid premature hypothyroidism and the worsening of eye disease. Those with severe conditions or significant changes in clinical manifestations should be closely observed as needed. After that, thyroid function monitoring should be performed every 4–8 weeks for up to half a year, or until the patient develops hypothyroidism and reaches a stable state after thyroid hormone replacement therapy. If complete remission is determined, the follow-up interval can be extended, and follow-up at least once a year is recommended [14].

Follow-up contents: (1) symptoms and signs; (2) laboratory tests: FT_3, FT_4 and TSH, and TRAb, TPOAb and TgAb can be tested if necessary and (3) for GD patients with complications; evaluation of the control of related disease symptoms and signs, and indicators changes should be noted.

11. Children and adolescents GD

GD accounts for about 95% of hyperthyroidism in children and adolescents. As a special group, they should be diagnosed and treated with great caution. There are great differences in treatment by different institutions and doctors. In addition to common clinical symptoms of GD, children may also be combined with decreased academic performance, inattention, anxiety, emotional instability, nervousness, hand tremor and active deep tendon reflexes [94]. In most countries, ATD is the preferred initial treatment for children and adolescents, but the relapse rate is high, with only 20–30% of patients achieving long-term remission after 2 years of ATD treatment [95]. Therefore, most children and adolescents with GD eventually need definitive treatment (RAI treatment or surgery).

If RAI is chosen to treat GD in children and adolescents, a sufficient single dose of RAI should be given to destroy the thyroid gland completely to achieve hypothyroidism. The goal of RAI treatment for GD is to induce hypothyroidism rather than euthyroidism, as a low RAI dose will result in residual and partially irradiated thyroid tissue, which may increase the risk of thyroid nodules and tumors [73, 96], and low dose has low remission rates. Therefore, to achieve hypothyroidism, RAI activity >150 μCi/g is necessary rather than a lower dose; for larger glands (50–80 g), RAI activity of 200–300 μCi/g or even higher may be necessary [97–99]. RAI should be avoided in very young children (<5 years). Children between 5 and 10 years of age can be treated with RAI if the activity >150 μCi/g and calculated RAI activity <10 mCi [5]. The therapeutic effect is related to gland size and dose [100], and thyroid hormone levels begin to decline within the first week after RAI treatment. The incidence of hypothyroidism in children treated with 50–100 μCi/g and 150–200 μCi/g was 20–45% and 60–95%, respectively [101–104]. Thyroid function should be monitored regularly after RAI treatment, and thyroid hormone replacement therapy should be initiated promptly if hypothyroidism occurs.

Other than the goal of hypothyroidism, side effects of RAI treatment in children and adolescents are uncommon. Less than 10% of children complain of mild thyroid tenderness within the first week after treatment, which can be managed symptomatically. Despite concerns about the safety of RAI treatment for children and adolescents and the potential for carcinogenesis and genetic damage [24], most studies consider that RAI treatment does not increase the risk of thyroid cancer, leukemia, or other cancers, or impaired fertility and increased rates of congenital malformations in offspring [5, 105–107]. Most children do not have a severe eye disease, and routine adjunctive prednisone therapy is not recommended. Nevertheless, prednisone (0.5 mg/kg for 4–6 weeks) may be beneficial for children and adolescents with moderate-to-severe eye disease who choose RAI treatment [99].

When choosing the treatment options for children and adolescents with GD, the theoretical risks of RAI must be weighed against thyroidectomy or long-term ATD use. The RAI activity should be based on the size and not be reduced arbitrarily because of the age of young adults. Attempting to minimize RAI activity may result in ineffectiveness, additional RAI treatment and radiation exposure. In conclusion, RAI treatment is a safe and definitive option for children and adolescents with GD.

12. Conclusion

RAI is an effective treatment for GD, especially for those who are ineffective to ATD treatment or have contraindications to surgery. For patients with severe symptoms or combined with cardiovascular disease and GO, the addition of β-adrenergic

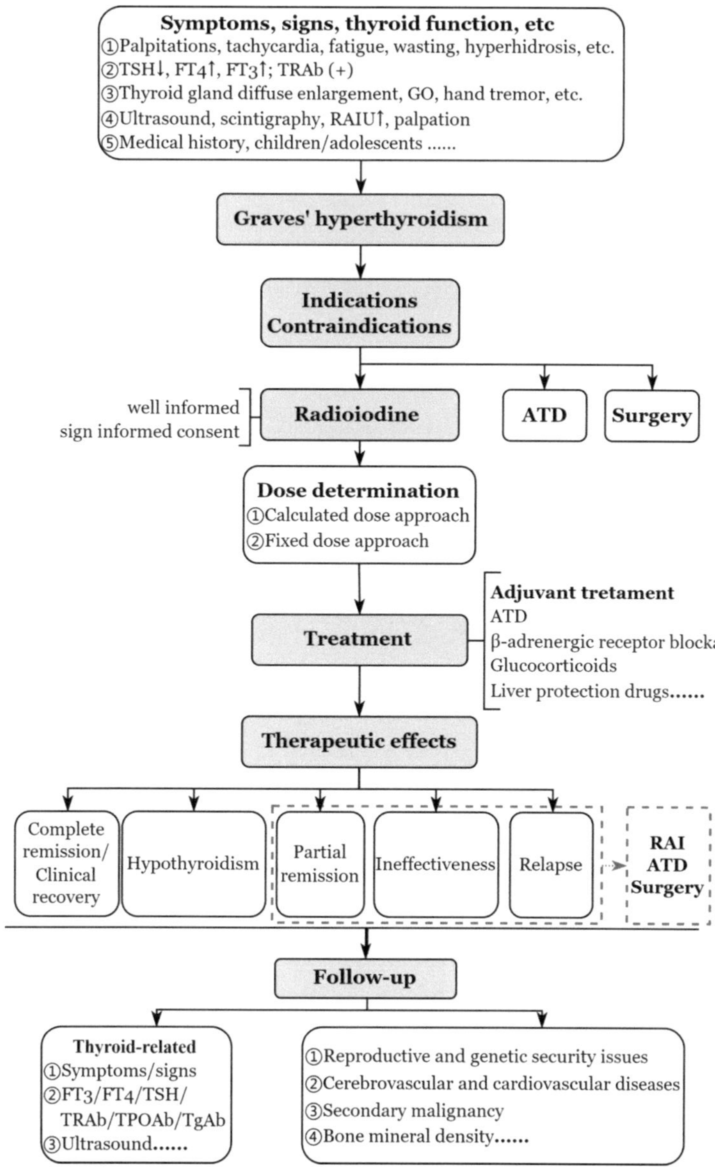

Figure 2.
General process of RAI treatment for GD.

blockade, ATD or glucocorticoids will effectively control the patient's condition. It is necessary to adjust the dose of RAI appropriately according to the patient's condition. Although there are many reports of side effects of RAI treatment for hyperthyroidism, mainly of those are all highly controversial. Overall, RAI is still a relatively safe treatment method and the general process is shown in **Figure 2**.

Conflict of interest

The authors declare no conflict of interest.

Author details

Yongji Jiang and Chao Ma*
Department of Nuclear Medicine, Shanghai Tenth People's Hospital, Tongji University School of Medicine, Shanghai, China

*Address all correspondence to: mc_7419@hotmail.com

References

[1] Bahn Chair RS, Burch HB, Cooper DS, Garber JR, Greenlee MC, Klein I, et al. Hyperthyroidism and other causes of thyrotoxicosis: Management guidelines of the American Thyroid Association and American Association of Clinical Endocrinologists. Thyroid. 2011;**21**(6):593-646

[2] Taylor PN, Albrecht D, Scholz A, Gutierrez-Buey G, Lazarus JH, Dayan CM. Global epidemiology of hyperthyroidism and hypothyroidism. Nature Reviews Endocrinology. 2018;**14**(5):301-316

[3] Villagelin D, Cooper DS, Burch HB. A 2023 international survey of clinical practice patterns in the management of Graves' disease: A decade of change. The Journal of Clinical Endocrinology and Metabolism. 2024:dgae222

[4] Kahaly GJ, Bartalena L, Hegedus L, Leenhardt L, Poppe K, Pearce SH. 2018 European Thyroid Association guideline for the management of Graves' hyperthyroidism. European Thyroid Journal. 2018;**7**(4):167-186

[5] Ross DS, Burch HB, Cooper DS, Greenlee MC, Laurberg P, Maia AL. 2016 American Thyroid Association guidelines for diagnosis and management of hyperthyroidism and other causes of thyrotoxicosis. Thyroid. 2016;**26**(10):1343-1421

[6] Parameswaran R, de Jong MC, Kit JLW, Sek K, Nam TQ, Thang TV. 2021 Asia-Pacific Graves' disease consortium survey of clinical practice patterns in the management of Graves' disease. Endocrine. 2023;**79**(1):135-142

[7] Burch HB, Burman KD, Cooper DS. A 2011 survey of clinical practice patterns in the management of Graves' disease. The Journal of Clinical Endocrinology and Metabolism. 2012;**97**(12):4549-4558

[8] Solomon B, Glinoer D, Lagasse R, Wartofsky L. Current trends in the management of Graves' disease. The Journal of Clinical Endocrinology and Metabolism. 1990;**70**(6):1518-1524

[9] Brito JP, Schilz S, Singh Ospina N, Rodriguez-Gutierrez R, Maraka S, Sangaralingham LR. Antithyroid drugs-the most common treatment for Graves' disease in the United States: A nationwide population-based study. Thyroid. 2016;**26**(8):1144-1145

[10] Chaker L, Cooper DS, Walsh JP, Peeters RP. Hyperthyroidism. The Lancet. 2024;**403**(10428):768-780

[11] Bonnema SJ, Hegedüs L. Radioiodine therapy in benign thyroid diseases: Effects, side effects, and factors affecting therapeutic outcome. Endocrine Reviews. 2012;**33**(6):920-980

[12] Kitahara CM, Berrington de Gonzalez A, Bouville A, Brill AB, Doody MM, Melo DR. Association of radioactive iodine treatment with cancer mortality in patients with hyperthyroidism. JAMA Internal Medicine. 2019;**179**(8):1034-1042

[13] la Cour JL, Jensen LT, Vej-Hansen A, Nygaard B. Radioiodine therapy increases the risk of cerebrovascular events in hyperthyroid and euthyroid patients. European Journal of Endocrinology. 2015;**172**(6):771-778

[14] Chinese Society of Nuclear Medicine. Clinical guidelines for ^{131}I treatment of Graves' hyperthyroidism (2021 edition).

Chinese Journal of Nuclear Medicine and Molecular Imaging. 2021;**41, 04**:242-253

[15] Klain M, Ricard M, Leboulleux S, Baudin E, Schlumberger M. Radioiodine therapy for papillary and follicular thyroid carcinoma. European Journal of Nuclear Medicine and Molecular Imaging. 2002;**29**(Suppl. 2):S479-S485

[16] Zhang R, Zhang G, Wang R, Tan J, He Y, Meng Z. Prediction of thyroidal ^{131}I effective half-life in patients with Graves' disease. Oncotarget. 2017;**8**(46):80934-80940

[17] Hautzel H, Pisar E, Yazdan-Doust N, Schott M, Beu M, Müller H-W. Qualitative and quantitative impact of protective glucocorticoid therapy on the effective ^{131}I half-life in radioiodine therapy for Graves disease. Journal of Nuclear Medicine. 2010;**51**(12):1917-1922

[18] Zakavi SR, Khazaei G, Sadeghi R, Ayati N, Davachi B, Bonakdaran S. Methimazole discontinuation before radioiodine therapy in patients with Graves' disease. Nuclear Medicine Communications. 2015;**36**(12):1202-1207

[19] Walter MA, Briel M, Christ-Crain M, Bonnema SJ, Connell J, Cooper DS. Effects of antithyroid drugs on radioiodine treatment: Systematic review and meta-analysis of randomised controlled trials. BMJ. 2007;**334**(7592):514

[20] Andrade VA, Gross JL, Maia AL. The effect of methimazole pretreatment on the efficacy of radioactive iodine therapy in Graves' hyperthyroidism: One-year follow-up of a prospective, randomized study. The Journal of Clinical Endocrinology and Metabolism. 2001;**86**(8):3488-3493

[21] Tagami T, Yambe Y, Tanaka T, Tanaka T, Ogo A, Yoshizumi H. Short-term effects of β-adrenergic antagonists and methimazole in new-onset thyrotoxicosis caused by Graves' disease. Internal Medicine. 2012;**51**(17):2285-2290

[22] Bartalena L, Baldeschi L, Boboridis K, Eckstein A, Kahaly GJ, Marcocci C. The 2016 European Thyroid Association/European Group on Graves' orbitopathy guidelines for the management of Graves' orbitopathy. European Thyroid Journal. 2016;**5**(1):9-26

[23] Davies TF, Andersen S, Latif R, Nagayama Y, Barbesino G, Brito M. Graves' disease. Nature Reviews Disease Primers. 2020;**6**(1):1-23

[24] Turcios S, Lence-Anta JJ, Santana J-L, Pereda CM, Velasco M, Chappe M. Thyroid volume and its relation to anthropometric measures in a healthy cuban population. European Thyroid Journal. 2015;**4**(1):55-61

[25] Wang H, Yu D, Tan Z, Hu R, Zhang B, Yu J. Estimation of thyroid volume from scintigraphy through 2D/3D registration of a statistical shape model. Physics in Medicine and Biology. 2019;**64**(9):095015

[26] Dottorini ME, Mansi L. Radioiodine in the management of benign thyroid disease: Clinical guidelines. In: Report of a Working Party, 2007. Royal College of Physicians (RCP). European Journal of Nuclear Medicine and Molecular Imaging. 2007;**12**(34):2148-2149

[27] Tamatea JA, Conaglen JV, Elston MS. Response to radioiodine therapy for thyrotoxicosis: Disparate outcomes for an indigenous population. International Journal of Endocrinology. 2016;**2016**(1):7863867

[28] Madu NM, Skinner C, Oyibo SO. Cure rates after a single dose of radioactive iodine to treat hyperthy

roidism: The fixed-dose regimen. Cureus;**14**(8):e28316

[29] Miller C, Al-Jabri A, O'Murchada L, Mustafa M, Cooke J, Phelan N. Use of a dosimetry-based RAI protocol for treatment of benign hyperthyroidism optimises response while minimising exposure to ionising radiation. Clinical Endocrinology. 2024;**100**(6):585-592

[30] Canto AU, Dominguez PN, Jimeno CA, Obaldo JM, Ogbac RV. Comparison of fixed versus calculated activity of radioiodine for the treatment of graves disease in adults. Endocrinology and Metabolism (Seoul). 2016;**31**(1):168-173

[31] January CT, Wann LS, Calkins H, Chen LY, Cigarroa JE, Cleveland JC Jr. 2019 AHA/ACC/HRS focused update of the 2014 AHA/ACC/HRS guideline for the management of patients with atrial fibrillation: A report of the American College of Cardiology/American Heart Association Task Force on Clinical Practice Guidelines and the Heart Rhythm Society in collaboration with the Society of Thoracic Surgeons. Circulation. 2019;**140**(2):e125-ee51

[32] Zhang Q, Guan Y, Xiang T, Liu S, Chen Q. Combination of molecular adsorbent recirculating system and radioiodine for the treatment of concurrent hyperthyroidism and severe liver dysfunction: A retrospective cohort study. Endocrine Practice. 2017;**23**(2):141-148

[33] Zhang Q, Zhang L, Xiang T, Guan Y, Liu S, Chen Q. A study on artificial liver system combined with ^{131}I in treatment of hyperthyroidism complicated by liver failure. Chinese Journal of Hepatology. 2016;**24**(10):778-782

[34] Yan D, Yu H, Yu G, Luo Q, Bao Y, Li L. Artificial liver support system combined with ^{131}I for severe jaundice caused by Grave's disease: A case report and literature review. Fudan University Journal of Medical Sciences. 2021;**48**(3):418-422

[35] Mumtaz M, Lin LS, Hui KC, Khir ASM. Radioiodine I-131 for the therapy of Graves' disease. The Malaysian Journal of Medical Sciences: MJMS. 2009;**16**(1):25

[36] Lee SY, Pearce EN. Hyperthyroidism: A review. Journal of the American Medical Association. 2023;**330**(15):1472-1483

[37] Perros P, Basu A, Boelaert K, Dayan C, Vaidya B, Williams GR. Postradioiodine Graves' management: The PRAGMA study. Clinical Endocrinology. 2022;**97**(5):664-675

[38] Fanning E, Inder WJ, Mackenzie E. Radioiodine treatment for graves' disease: A 10-year Australian cohort study. BMC Endocrine Disorders. 2018;**18**(1):94

[39] Stan MN, Durski JM, Brito JP, Bhagra S, Thapa P, Bahn RS. Cohort study on radioactive iodine–induced hypothyroidism: Implications for Graves' ophthalmopathy and optimal timing for thyroid hormone assessment. Thyroid. 2013;**23**(5):620-625

[40] Nygaard B, Hegedus L, Gervil M, Hjalgrim H, Hansen BM, Soe-Jensen P. Influence of compensated radioiodine therapy on thyroid volume and incidence of hypothyroidism in Graves' disease. Journal of Internal Medicine. 1995;**238**(6):491-497

[41] Knapska-Kucharska M, Oszukowska L, Lewiński A. Analysis of demographic and clinical factors affecting the outcome of adioiodine therapy in patients with hyperthyroidism. Archives of Medical Science. 2010;**6**(4):611-622

[42] Šfiligoj D, Gaberšcek S, Mekjavic PJ, Pirnat E, Zaletel K. Factors influencing the success of radioiodine therapy in patients with Graves' disease. Nuclear Medicine Communications. 2015;**36**(6):560-565

[43] Li JF, Xie LJ, Qin LP, Wan QC, Li JP, Wu QY. Development of hypothyroidism over 13 years of follow-up of patients with hyperthyroidism after radioiodine therapy. Hellenic Journal of Nuclear Medicine. 2022;**25**(1):26-31

[44] Li J, Zhang L, Zhang Z, Liu J, Zhang H, Lin X. Factors suggesting relapse of Grave's disease after first radioiodine therapy. Analysis of 607 cases. Hellenic Journal of Nuclear Medicine. 2019;**22**(1):64-69

[45] Wiersinga WM. Graves' disease: Can it be cured? Endocrinology and Metabolism. 2019;**34**(1):29-38

[46] Yang Y-T, Chen J-F, Tung S-C, Kuo M-C, Weng S-W, Chou C-K. Long-term outcome and prognostic factors of single-dose Radioiodine Therapy in patients with Graves' disease. Journal of the Formosan Medical Association. 2020;**119**(5):925-932

[47] Xing Y-Z, Zhang K, Jin G. Predictive factors for the outcomes of Graves' disease patients with radioactive iodine (^{131}I) treatment. Bioscience Reports. 2020;**40**(1):BSR20191609

[48] Yang D, Xue J, Ma W, Liu F, Fan Y, Rong J. Prognostic factor analysis in 325 patients with Graves' disease treated with radioiodine therapy. Nuclear Medicine Communications. 2018;**39**(1):16-21

[49] Szumowski P, Abdelrazek S, Sawicka AK, Mojsak M, Kostecki J, Sykała M. Radioiodine therapy for Graves' disease—Retrospective analysis of efficacy factors. Endokrynologia Polska. 2015;**66**(2):126-131

[50] Plazinska MT, Sawicka-Gutaj N, Czarnywojtek A, Wolinski K, Kobylecka M, Karlinska M. Radioiodine therapy and Graves' disease—Myths and reality. PLoS ONE. 2020;**15**(1):e0226495

[51] Quataert F, Bravenboer B, Keyaerts M, Andreescu CE. The presence of anti-TPO antibodies increase the likelihood of post-I131 hypothyroidism. Hormone and Metabolic Research. 2024;**56**(2):134-141

[52] Sapienza MT, Coura-Filho GB, Willegaignon J, Watanabe T, Duarte PS, Buchpiguel CA. Clinical and dosimetric variables related to outcome after treatment of Graves' disease with 550 and 1110 MBq of ^{131}I: Results of a prospective randomized trial. Clinical Nuclear Medicine. 2015;**40**(9):715-719

[53] Khan MSA, Hussain A, Ahmad S, Shah MH. Outcomes of radioactive iodine (^{131}I) therapy among hyperthyroid patients. Pakistan Journal of Medical Sciences. 2023;**39**(6):1685

[54] Saadat N, Azizi F, Abdi H, Amouzegar A. Treatment of post-radioactive iodine relapse of hyperthyroidism: Comparison of long-term methimazole and radioactive iodine treatment. Journal of Endocrinological Investigation. 2022;**45**(10):1919-1924

[55] Bartalena L, Piantanida E, Gallo D, Lai A, Tanda ML. Epidemiology, natural history, risk factors, and prevention of Graves' orbitopathy. Frontiers in Endocrinology. 2020;**11**:615993

[56] Burch HB, Wartofsky L. Graves' ophthalmopathy: Current concepts regarding pathogenesis and management. Endocrine Reviews. 1993;**14**(6):747-793

[57] Ma C, Xie J, Wang H, Li J, Chen S. Radioiodine therapy versus antithyroid medications for Graves' disease.

Cochrane Database of Systematic Reviews. 2016;**2**(2):Cd010094

[58] Traisk F, Tallstedt L, Abraham-Nordling M, Andersson T, Berg G, Calissendorff J. Thyroid-associated ophthalmopathy after treatment for Graves' hyperthyroidism with antithyroid drugs or iodine-131. The Journal of Clinical Endocrinology and Metabolism. 2009;**94**(10):3700-3707

[59] Watanabe N, Noh JY, Kozaki A, Iwaku K, Sekiya K, Kosuga Y. Radioiodine-associated exacerbation of Graves' orbitopathy in the Japanese population: Randomized prospective study. The Journal of Clinical Endocrinology and Metabolism. 2015;**100**(7):2700-2708

[60] Bartalena L, Tanda ML. Current concepts regarding Graves' orbitopathy. Journal of Internal Medicine. 2022;**292**(5):692-716

[61] Hussain F, Adil M, Hussain M. Radioactive iodine therapy for hyperthyroidism. In: Hyperthyroidism-Recent Updates. London, UK: IntechOpen; 2023

[62] Liu X, Wong CKH, Wu T, Chan WWL, Woo YC, Lam CLK. A comparison of cardiovascular disease, cancer, mortality, and Graves' ophthalmopathy following treatment for hyperthyroidism: A Bayesian network meta-analysis. World Journal of Surgery. 2024;**48**(2):393-407

[63] Stein JD, Childers D, Gupta S, Talwar N, Nan B, Lee BJ. Risk factors for developing thyroid-associated ophthalmopathy among individuals with Graves disease. JAMA Ophthalmology. 2015;**133**(3):290-296

[64] Khiyani N, Dadparvar S, Gish A, Intenzo CM, Malmud LS. Does the dose of iodine-131 influence the incidence of Graves' ophthalmopathy? Nuclear Medicine Communications. 2019;**40**(5):455-460

[65] Oculoplastic and Orbital Disease Group of Chinese Ophthalmological Society of Chinese Medical Association, Thyroid Group of Chinese Society of Endocrinology of Chinese Medical Association. Guidelines for diagnosis and management of hyperthyroidism and other causes of thyrotoxicosis. Chinese Journal of Endocrinology and Metabolism. 2022;**2022**(09):646-668

[66] Vannucchi G, Covelli D, Campi I, Currò N, Dazzi D, Rodari M. Prevention of orbitopathy by oral or intravenous steroid prophylaxis in short duration Graves' disease patients undergoing radioiodine ablation: A prospective randomized control trial study. Thyroid. 2019;**29**(12):1828-1833

[67] Shiber S, Stiebel-Kalish H, Shimon I, Grossman A, Robenshtok E. Glucocorticoid regimens for prevention of Graves' ophthalmopathy progression following radioiodine treatment: Systematic review and meta-analysis. Thyroid. 2014;**24**(10):1515-1523

[68] Prummel MF, Wiersinga WM, Mourits MP, Koornneef L, Berghout A, van der Gaag R. Effect of abnormal thyroid function on the severity of Graves' ophthalmopathy. Archives of Internal Medicine. 1990;**150**(5):1098-1101

[69] Kahaly GJ. Imaging in thyroid-associated orbitopathy. European Journal of Endocrinology. 2001;**145**(2):107-118

[70] Wang R, Tan J, Zhang G, Long L. The effect of ^{99}Tc-methylene diphosphonate on Graves ophthalmopathy treated by ^{131}I. Chinese Journal of Postgraduates of Medicine. 2009;**12**:27-29

[71] Marcocci C, Kahaly GJ, Krassas GE, Bartalena L, Prummel M, Stahl M. Selenium and the course of mild Graves' orbitopathy. New England Journal of Medicine. 2011;**364**(20):1920-1931

[72] Saenger EL, Thoma GE, Tompkins EA. Incidence of leukemia following treatment of hyperthyroidism. Preliminary report of the Cooperative Thyrotoxicosis Therapy Follow-Up Study. Journal of the American Medical Association. 1968;**205**(12):855-862

[73] Dobyns BM, Sheline GE, Workman JB, Tompkins EA, McConahey WM, Becker DV. Malignant and benign neoplasms of the thyroid in patients treated for hyperthyroidism: A report of the cooperative thyrotoxicosis therapy follow-up study. The Journal of Clinical Endocrinology and Metabolism. 1974;**38**(6):976-998

[74] Ron E, Doody MM, Becker DV, Brill AB, Curtis RE, Goldman MB. Cancer mortality following treatment for adult hyperthyroidism. Cooperative Thyrotoxicosis Therapy Follow-up Study Group. Journal of the American Medical Association. 1998;**280**(4):347-355

[75] Vasileiou M, Gilbert J, Fishburn S, Boelaert K, Guideline C. Thyroid disease assessment and management: Summary of NICE guidance. BMJ. 2020;**368**:m41

[76] Gronich N, Lavi I, Rennert G, Saliba W. Cancer risk after radioactive iodine treatment for hyperthyroidism: A cohort study. Thyroid. 2020;**30**(2):243-250

[77] Boelaert K, Maisonneuve P, Torlinska B, Franklyn JA. Comparison of mortality in hyperthyroidism during periods of treatment with thionamides and after radioiodine. The Journal of Clinical Endocrinology and Metabolism. 2013;**98**(5):1869-1882

[78] Hindié E, Ain KB, Zerdoud S, Avram AM. Association of radioactive iodine treatment of hyperthyroidism with cancer mortality: An unjustified warning? The Journal of Clinical Endocrinology and Metabolism. 2020;**105**(4):e1901-e19e2

[79] Franklyn JA, Maisonneuve P, Sheppard M, Betteridge J, Boyle P. Cancer incidence and mortality after radioiodine treatment for hyperthyroidism: A population-based cohort study. Lancet. 1999;**353**(9170):2111-2115

[80] Hall P, Berg G, Bjelkengren G, Boice JD Jr, Ericsson UB, Hallquist A. Cancer mortality after iodine-131 therapy for hyperthyroidism. International Journal of Cancer. 1992;**50**(6):886-890

[81] Metso S, Auvinen A, Huhtala H, Salmi J, Oksala H, Jaatinen P. Increased cancer incidence after radioiodine treatment for hyperthyroidism. Cancer. 2007;**109**(10):1972-1979

[82] Holm LE, Hall P, Wiklund K, Lundell G, Berg G, Bjelkengren G. Cancer risk after iodine-131 therapy for hyperthyroidism. Journal of the National Cancer Institute. 1991;**83**(15):1072-1077

[83] La Cour JL, Andersen UB, Sørensen CH, Nygaard B, Jensen LT. Radioiodine therapy does not change the atherosclerotic burden of the carotid arteries. Thyroid. 2016;**26**(7):965-971

[84] Giesecke P, Frykman V, Wallin G, Lonn S, Discacciati A, Torring O. All-cause and cardiovascular mortality risk after surgery versus radioiodine treatment for hyperthyroidism. The British Journal of Surgery. 2018;**105**(3):279-286

[85] Peng CC-H, Lin Y-J, Lee SY, Lin S-M, Han C, Loh C-H. MACE and hyperthyroidism treated with

medication, radioactive iodine, or thyroidectomy. JAMA Network Open. 2024;**7**(3):e240904-e

[86] Liu X, Wong CK, Chan WW, Tang EH, Woo YC, Lam CL. Outcomes of Graves' disease patients following antithyroid drugs, radioactive iodine, or thyroidectomy as the first-line treatment. Annals of Surgery. 2021;**273**(6):1197-1206

[87] Graham GD, Burman KD. Radioiodine treatment of Graves' disease: An assessment of its potential risks. Annals of Internal Medicine. 1986;**105**(6):900-905

[88] Liu L, Liu B, Huang R, Kuang A. Radiation protection and safety in nuclear medicine. Chinese Journal of Medical Imaging Technology. 2017;**33**(12):1888-1892

[89] Ceccarelli C, Canale D, Battisti P, Caglieresi C, Moschini C, Fiore E. Testicular function after ^{131}I therapy for hyperthyroidism. Clinical Endocrinology. 2006;**65**(4):446-452

[90] Zhang LH, Li JY, Tian Q, Liu S, Zhang H, Liu S. Follow-up and evaluation of the pregnancy outcome in women of reproductive age with Graves' disease after ^{131}Iodine treatment. Journal of Radiation Research. 2016;**57**(6):702-708

[91] Guan L, Chen G, Zhang J, Wang L. The preliminary clinical observation and analysis of childbearingage women with a history of iodine-131 treatment for Graves' disease. Bioscience Trends. 2016;**10**(4):307-314

[92] Ohrling H, Torring O, Yin L, Iliadou AN, Tullgren O, Abraham-Nordling M. Decreased birth weight, length, and head circumference in children born by women years after treatment for hyperthyroidism. The Journal of Clinical Endocrinology and Metabolism. 2014;**99**(9):3217-3223

[93] Mattsson S, Bernhardsson C. Release of patients after radionuclide therapy: Radionuclide releases to the environment from hospitals and patients. In: Radiation Protection in Nuclear Medicine. Berlin, Heidelberg: Springer; 2012. pp. 139-148

[94] Vaidyanathan P. Update on pediatric hyperthyroidism. Advances in Pediatrics. 2022;**69**(1):219-229

[95] Léger J, Carel JC. Diagnosis and management of hyperthyroidism from prenatal life to adolescence. Best Practice & Research Clinical Endocrinology & Metabolism. 2018;**32**(4):373-386

[96] Ron E, Lubin JH, Shore RE, Mabuchi K, Modan B, Pottern LM. Thyroid cancer after exposure to external radiation: A pooled analysis of seven studies. Radiation Research. 1995;**141**(3):259-277

[97] Rivkees SA, Cornelius EA. Influence of iodine-131 dose on the outcome of hyperthyroidism in children. Pediatrics. 2003;**111**(4):745-749

[98] Rivkees SA, Dinauer C. An optimal treatment for pediatric Graves' disease is radioiodine. The Journal of Clinical Endocrinology and Metabolism. 2007;**92**(3):797-800

[99] Rivkees SA. Approach to the patient: Management and the long-term consequences of Graves' disease in children. The Journal of Clinical Endocrinology and Metabolism. 2022;**107**(12):3408-3417

[100] Sheremeta M, Korchagina M, Trukhin A, Nagaeva E, Bezlepkina O, Peterkova V. Thyroid volume is the key predictor of hyperthyroidism remission

after radioactive iodine therapy in pediatric patients. European Journal of Pediatrics. 2023;**182**(11):4931-4937

[101] Glaser NS, Styne DM, Organization of Pediatric Endocrinologists of Northern California Collaborative Graves' Disease Study Group. Predicting the likelihood of remission in children with Graves' disease: A prospective, multicenter study. Pediatrics. 2008;**121**(3):e481-e4e8

[102] Azizi F, Amouzegar A. Management of thyrotoxicosis in children and adolescents: 35 years' experience in 304 patients. Journal of Pediatric Endocrinology and Metabolism. 2018;**31**(2):159-165

[103] Rivkees SA, Sklar C, Freemark M. The management of Graves' disease in children, with special emphasis on radioiodine treatment. The Journal of Clinical Endocrinology and Metabolism. 1998;**83**(11):3767-3776

[104] Ballal S, Soundararajan R, Singh H, Garg A, Chopra S, Bal C. Influence of prior carbimazole on the outcome of radioiodine therapy in pediatric and adolescent Graves' disease. Nuclear Medicine Communications. 2015;**36**(6):566-572

[105] Lutterman SL, Zwaveling-Soonawala N, Verberne HJ, Verburg FA, van Trotsenburg ASP, Mooij CF. The efficacy and short- and long-term side effects of radioactive iodine treatment in pediatric Graves' disease: A systematic review. European Thyroid Journal. 2021;**10**(5):353-363

[106] Read CH Jr, Tansey MJ, Menda Y. A 36-year retrospective analysis of the efficacy and safety of radioactive iodine in treating young Graves' patients. The Journal of Clinical Endocrinology and Metabolism. 2004;**89**(9):4229-4233

[107] Mooij CF, Cheetham TD, Verburg FA, Eckstein A, Pearce SH, Léger J. 2022 European Thyroid Association Guideline for the management of pediatric Graves' disease. European Thyroid Journal. 2022;**11**(1):e210073